C000047538

THE OTHER SIDE *of* ONA

MEGAN M. TERABERRY

A'o Nīnaus II

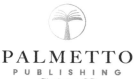

PALMETTO
P U B L I S H I N G
Charleston, SC
www.PalmettoPublishing.com

Copyright © 2024 by Megan M Teraberry

All rights reserved
No portion of this book may be reproduced, stored in a retrieval system, or transmitted in any form by any means–electronic, mechanical,
photocopy, recording, or other–except for brief quotations in printed
reviews, without prior permission of the author.

First Edition

Hardcover: 979-8-8229-3856-4
Paperback: 979-8-8229-3857-1
eBook: 979-8-8229-4056-7

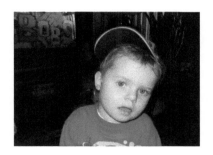

This book I dedicate to my dear beloved son:
Damien Carter Layton.
Who has inspired me in so many ways then I
could ever express, in a
 life time.No amount of words or
Actions could hardly be said or even begin to
be written about how
 much he has inspired me.
Let alone taught me to be the best mother I
can be for my
daughter! I will forever love You and miss you,
fly safe my sweet
 angel boy. You are missed by so many.
Your story Lives on, your smile as promised
won't be forgotten
 and nor will your laugh. 3/8/2006
—10/18/2011

Boise you're the best: Blue and true:

Boise peeps I wanted to personally drop you all a line this time! I'd like to personally thank you all for your love, support, and all that you not only do for me, but also for our lovely community! Without you this place wouldn't be as whole or complete.

Whether we are enjoying the trails for a hike, fishing outdoors, gardening, motorcycle rides, or enjoying time indoors as a community, regardless of what beverages we may be having, I love how as a community we get together and enjoy life no matter what is going on! Boise you have been a wonderful bright spot in my life and have taught me so much. Thank you. My hope to you is that this will bring you joy and inspiration too! Love you all always!

I love how we all look out for those silly ducks and geese that like to cross; well, you guys know, the streets. They sure are precious to us yet, I'm sure, annoy the visitors, lol. jk. Definitely don't be in a hurry when the geese/ducks are crossing here! I also love how as a community we are so forgiving, loving, kind, wholesome, and we all get together when there is a need. I honestly gotta say that I found a home within a home, a love within a love, and a life I didn't think was possible, and I have Boise to thank for that—so, thank you.

So very many Dreams do come true!

NEW?

- Why do things have to itch?

- Why is the world round?

- What is the shape of the universe?

- Does the universe have a shape?

- Why does it take babies so long to learn to talk?

- What was your favorite kids' story and fairytale?

- What is the difference between a story and a fairytale?

- Do you like pain?

- Why do we want what others have?

- How many MRIs are there?

– Why does pollen attract bees?

– What makes honey so sweet?

– Do you believe in reincarnation?

– What would you come back as?

– What do you support?

– Do you write down your thoughts?

– What do you consider as a corner?

– How many exits are there?

– How many windows are there?

– Are the eyes really the windows to the soul?

– How many lights are there?

– Breakfast or dinner?

– How long will we all have to wear masks for?

- Will the universe clear the air?

- How much oxygen do we breathe in a day?

- How many brains are there?

- Would you rather be patient or be a patient?

- How much tolerance do you have?

- How many people have blond, black, grey and red hair?

- How many hair colors are there?

- How many different sounds can birds make?

- Do you like watching TV?

- What would you rather be doing right now?

- How many technical difficulties are there in a day?

- How long can you go without caffeine?

- Do you have a pacemaker?

- Have you ever had your heart stop?

- Would you give a ride to a stranger?

- What's the longest that you've ever cried?

- Do you remember how you learned how to draw a flower?

- How many sweats do you have?

- Who do you think about throughout the day and night?

- What's the most watched tv show?

- What is the most bought piece of clothing?

- What are you making in your life?

- If one is productive, can they also be depressed?

- What are some of your reminders in your life?

- Who's been your training wheels in your life?

- Who's trying to stop you from success/succeeding?

- How do you save money?

- What's the best way to save money?

- What's a good investment?

- Do you invest in yourself?

- Do you have birds that whisper in your ear?

- Were you a happy little accident?

- Do you ever think of how much your life could change so much over time?

- How real are you?

- How much gets posted on the internet in a day?

- How much is going on?

- How much is too much to get done?

- Where will they attack next?

- What are ants after?

- What is the most annoying bug?

- Is science in a way its own language?

- Are you secure?

- Are we, you confident?

- Can you go it alone?

- How lonely is lonely?

- Can you hear your own thoughts?

- How do you escape?

– Where is the best place to hide?

– Where is the best place to be?

– What are you finishing up?

– What is your experience?

– How many gears are there?

– What drives you?

– What is consistent?

– Do you have will power?

– What's the best romance story?

– What changed your mind?

– How is it that at times of our lives we think we know everything and yet we know nothing?

– Have you ever started over?

– What do you eat?

– Have you ever been engaged?

– What is the craziest story ever told?

– Are you cursed?

– How many curses are there?

– How many people do you know in your family?

– If the human race ended what kind of connection would be left?

– Would you save the human race?

– Do you have muscles?

– How many muscles are there?

– How does one do their work with a smile every day?

– Can you predict the future?

– Do you have visions?

– Do your visions come true?

- Is reality just an illusion?

- How much will I get done?

- What's the most annoying animal?

- Have you gotten to know yourself?

- How much writing is there?

- How many dolls are there?

- How many snow globes are there?

- Do spells really work?

- What do you consider to be witchcraft?

- Who would you think is a witch?

- What do you aspire to be?

- Is sleep considered a chore?

- How are chores defined?

- Who decides what's a chore?

- How many chores are there?

- Do you have a rain stick?

- What's that look for?

- What do you look up?

- What's your favorite thing to research?

- Who do you want?

- What's taking so long?

- How long does it take you to finish something?

- What things have you accomplished today?

- What are you hooked on?

- What's your magic?

- What are you grateful for?

- What do you wish?

- Do you know what day it is?

- What have you wasted time on?

- Have you ever been left with bad directions?

- Have you ever reminisced about the past?

- If you were without power for a week, would you be prepared?

- What's the craziest movie ever made?

- Does anybody ever get a hold of you?

- What is the most cooked dish?

- What is the most wanted food?

- Have you ever split wood?

- How many smiles are there?

- Do you ever think or feel like you're being invaded?

– What does alien stand for?

– What are you willing to go through?

– What was I just looking at?

– How long is the longest thing?

– Would you take a shot before you died?

– Have you ever shot a gun?

– Have you ever been hunting?

– Why does one have to go up to get down and down to get up?

– Have you ever listened to the rain?

– Have you ever listened to the snow?

– Does a rainbow have any sound?

– How many lessons are there in life?

– Are there lessons after death?

- Why is incense so calming?

- Why are some attracted to fire?

- Why are there only four elements?

- If there were more elements would love or light be one of them?

- Why are there only seven chakras?

- How long does it take to get to enlightenment?

- Do you follow suggestions?

- What path have you chosen?

- How many paths are there?

- At what point does one grow up?

- Is God real and if so, how real?

- What music makes you move?

- How do you do you?

– Do you ever tell people things that you wish they would tell you?

– Can I do ten pages a day?

– How many journals are there?

– How many journals become books?

– What's your broken glass?

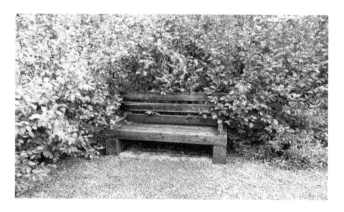

– What is symbolic?

– Where do you belong?

– Have you ever been in the dark?

– What do you like to look at?

– What are your temptations?

– Have you ever learned martial arts?

– How many wedding dresses are there?

– What lowers your standards?

– How many weddings are performed?

– How many comics are there?

– Where would you move to?

– What is abstract in your life?

– Why are there tiny lights in a well-lit room?

– Are you good at hiding or is anyone even looking?

– Have you realized that it's been you the whole time?

– How many realizations are there?

– How many buildings are there?

– What kind of schedule do you have?

– What does peace look like?

– How many signs are there?

– How much pain is too much?

– Where did you get your ink done?

– Have you ever read a comic book?

– How many comic books are there?

– How does an hour feel?

– Have you ever been in a limo?

– What is limbo?

– How many get struck by lightning?

– Who do you hear from?

– What's your story line?

- How do you write an ending?

- Can you listen to your thoughts?

- Can you sit in silence and if so, how long?

- Would you do a documentary on you?

- Do you stay dry when it rains, or do you dance in it?

- How can you tell something is real or fake?

- What is your music like?

- How many clouds go by in a day?

- How many blankets are there?

- Where's the best place to write a book?

- How many new things are made let alone created in a day?

– What's the best analogy?

– What's the best phrase?

– What is the difference between analogy and a phrase?

– How many people cry in a day?

– How much coffee is there?

– What are all of the different kinds of coffees?

– Would you reach out even if you didn't want to?

– Have you ever broken a promise?

– How many promises are there?

– What would you do to keep your sanity?

– Are you afraid to feel?

– How many feelings do you feel in a day?

- Do you share?

- How do you show care?

- Have you tasted blood?

- How true are the Grimm stories?

- What stories do you tell?

- How many stories are there?

- Do you believe in magic?

- Do you know your family crest?

- What is heritage to you?

- What is the one thing that always feeds the soul?

- Have you bought enough art?

- What is considered art?

- How many categories are there?

- What happens to all of the test results over the years?

- How many planets have disappeared?

- How many stars disappear?

- Do you have nick names for your Neighbors?

- What jokes do you know?

- How much gets covered up?

- What smell would you want to smell?

- How many smells are there?

- Is there a place of peace?

- What is pain to you?

- How many people really understand what they are reading?

- What is going on?

- Do you like to get your nails done?

- What places have you gone to?

- What are your favorite places of business to go?

- Do you like to exercise?

- What colors have you had your nails painted?

- Have you ever been to a spa?

- How many spas are there?

- What is considered a spa?

- How many water bottles are there?

- How many water bottles do you have?

- Do you reuse items in your life?

- What things can you make/create?

- How many chairs are there?

- How many things get thrown out on a daily basis?

- How much is too much?

- Do you pay for what you get?

- Why are somethings overpriced and others underpriced?

- Have you ever been rock climbing?

- What is ideal to you?

- How much tv do you watch?

- What does exercise do for you?

- Do you smile for the picture?

- Are you okay with your mistakes?

- Do you get pretty for you or someone else?

- How much caffeine do you have?

- How many vitamins are there?

- How are vitamins considered to be vitamins?

- What would people do if they had nothing to complain about?

- How fast can you walk?

- What's the slowest walk?

- How many people have you talked with in a day?

- How much water do you have in a day?

- What triggers your mood?

- What brings up you're stress levels?

- Can you talk to anyone?

- What is your dream job?

- Have you ever been a standup comedian?

- Where's your head at?

- Have you ever counted grains of sand?

- Do you own a suite?

- Why do we settle?

- Why do we let ourselves down?

- What are accomplishments to you?

- Where have you found love?

- What are you connected to?

- What does connection mean to you?

- What mystery is in your life?

- What is mysterious to you?

- Why is mystery so intriguing?

- What keeps mystery alive?

- Why lies in your fears?

- What creates a fear?

- How did gears come about?

- What was the first scary story told?

- What scary stories have you been told?

- What's the difference between a story and a fairytale?

- How do you become enlightened?

- How much blood is on the ground let alone in the soil?

- How much blood is lost in a lifetime and where does it go?

- How much do you know?

- What is real to you?

- Who are you thankful for?

- Have you ever done a list of gratitudes?

– How many conversations can you listen to all at once?

– How many hot springs are there?

– are there any hot springs that have not been found yet?

– How many sentences are there?

– Have you ever felt trapped?

– How many times have you settled?

– Have you ever been behind a door that you felt you couldn't open?

– Have you ever been talked off the ledge before?

– Does it hurt?

– How much pain can you endure?

– What do you feel like?

– Where do you think of?

- What sets you off?

- What is the loudest noise?

- Who do you trust?

- Do you trust yourself?

- What do you feel?

- What is the brightest light?

- What would you have done differently?

- What changes are you making in your life?

- Are you growing?

- What's your favorite food?

- Are you artistic?

- What sparks your memory?

- How do you get past traumas?

– How much trauma have you been through?

– What is your main focus?

– Can you let go?

– What are you holding onto?

– What does crazy look like to you?

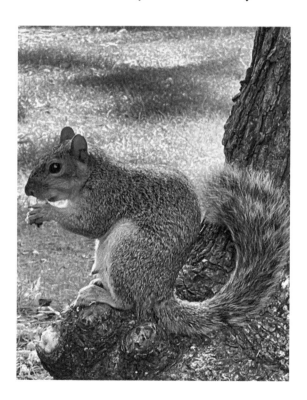

– What time is it?

– How heartless have you become?

– What colors inspire you?

– What colors are too bright for you?

– Would you let you down?

– Have you ever people watched?

– What's the most time you've put into something?

– Can you sing?

– Are you where you want to be?

– What's stopping you?

– Are you comfortable?

– Do you smell good when you sweat?

– Did you talk to God today?

– How do you help people like me?

- How well do you handle death?

- What do you do for Mother Earth?

- What's the last thing you did for yourself?

- Can you afford a truck?

- Do you give to charity?

- What is clarity to you?

- How do you sneeze?

- How much paperwork do you do?

- Where do you stand?

- How much do you hear?

- How much do you speak?

- What sparks your interest?

- What are your hobbies?

- What do you like to think about?

- What do you save for later?

- How many lies do you tell yourself?

- What do you contribute to?

- Who do you know?

- Are you who you think you are?

- Where should you be?

- How much do you do in a day?

- What do you visualize?

- How many questions fit on ten pages?

- Where are your truths?

- How long do you hold things in?

- How do you relax?

- How many parks are there?

- Have you ever read upside down?

– Do you have a purpose?

– What is balance to you?

– Are the questions really the story?

– How many questions are in a movie?

– What are you growing?

– What have you grown?

– What makes you thirsty?

– What torchers you?

– Have you had a date with the opposite sex?

– Do you have an art journal?

– How do you meditate?

– What skin care do you do?

– What is your sexual orientation?

- How long is the longest
  conversation?

- What's the best date?

- Have you ever been proposed to?

- Have you ever proposed?

- How many people support you?

- Do you support you?

- What's your favorite drama?

- What would you get rid of in your
  life?

- Would you move for someone?

- Are you ok?

- What do wish you could take back?

- What should be done?

- What's something you would give up
  for someone else?

- Are you desperate?

- Are you, someone else's desperation?

- What inspires you?

- Do all scales measure the same?

- Whose opinion matters the most?

- Do you go to old, sorted places and reminisce?

- How do you hide your emotions?

- Would you tell on yourself?

- How good are you?

- How bad is bad?

- Who's your fantasy?

- Do you know yourself?

- How many corrections are there?

- What stimulates you?

– What's your favorite drink?

– What's the earliest you've been to an appointment?

– How many doctors do you see?

– How much does outside help cost?

– How many trees are there?

– How many gates are there?

– Do you put up a wall?

– How guarded are you?

– Are you okay with making mistakes?

– What have you learned in the last year?

– Would you share even if it was, your last....?

– Have you ever had an out of body experience?

– What is truth?

– Are you deceiving yourself?

– What is considered art?

– Are you creative?

– Who's the fastest typer?

– How many texts are sent in a day?

– Are we Gods entertainment?

– What's grounded?

– What does fall in peace mean to you?

– How many windows are there?

– What's holding you back?

– What have you created?

– What's the most sought-after color?

– Who would you donate to?

– Can I just pack up and leave?

– Have you ever left?

– What do you feel guilty about?

– Do cats sweat?

– Who do you want to be?

– Do you want to be you?

– Have you ever given a speech?

– Have you gone crazy?

– How many symptoms are there?

– Have you ever been watched?

– How well do you know yourself?

– What pains you?

– How many dresses are there?

– Does tastes inspire?

- What is your fantasy?

- What's the weirdest outfit that you've ever worn?

- Does change ever make anyone else feel like a failure?

- Are you afraid to move forward?

- What do you feel like after you finish your goals?

- What embarrassing things have happened to you?

- Have you ever felt like ripping something out of your body?

- Do you ever feel like crawling into a ball and crying?

- What are you working on?

- What Aw ha moments have overturned your life?

- Have you settled?

- Are you where you want to be now?

- Are you doing what you love?

- How honest are you?

- What lies do you tell yourself?

- How wild can you run?

- Do you like camping?

- What is your story?

- What are you gossiping about?

- Who have you left behind?

- Have you broken any hearts?

- Do you listen to yourself or others?

- Who do you side with?

- What is deeper the ocean or human thought?

- How do you look upside down?

– Is going or growing better?

– Do you support what you do and how?

– Do you want to go?

– Do you want to play with me?

– What is your favorite character to play?

– Do you like to dress up?

– Do you like games?

– Are there as many stars as there are sentences?

– How many broken hearts are there?

– Have you realized yet you are the master of what?

– What is life to you in a world full of chaos?

– What do you color with?

– What hats do you like?

– Smooth or rough?

– Calm or wild?

– How do you feel about reflections?

– Closets or dressers?

– Dark or light?

– Sunset or sunrise?

– What's the most appealing time of day?

– What's the most appealing time of night?

– Why is the full moon so sought after?

– What is blissful to you?

– Where do the hands of time turn best for you?

– What beat of music gets you moving to the Rhythm of your heartbeat?

– Do you like to dance?

– Will travels suite you?

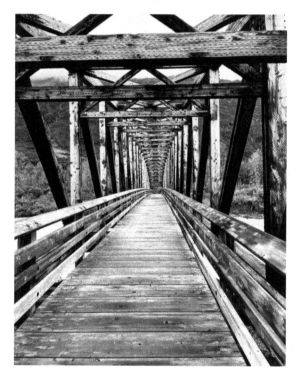

– Where shall we travel to?

– What is your crush?

- Where would you dream of being at?

- What does peace of mind mean to you?

- Would you get matching tattoos?

- How many times have you fallen?

- How courageous are you?

- How does God feel?

- Does God have a heartbeat?

- Is there time in space?

- Where does our breath go?

- Does the soul die?

- What lights your flame?

- What's got you spinning?

- Do you compliment people?

- How well do you handle a compliment or a complaint?

- What sad story do you know?

- What is up lifting?

- Does God cry?

- Can the devil catch feelings?

- Can you start over?

- How many things have you gotten out of?

- How many crazy things happen in a day?

- What does silence do for you?

- How are you going to accomplish your goals?

- What scares you the most?

- How are some still alive and others have died?

- Do you have a strong will to live?

- Who are you waiting for?

- Are you appreciated?

- What's the most important thing to you?

- What's a few minutes to you?

- Do you have any children?

- If you could ask one question to the whole world, what would it be?

- I love you, but do you love me?

- How many circles are there?

- What have you figured out?

- How many schools are there?

- How much food is there?

- Do you like rainbows?

– Are you easily distracted?

– Are you trapped?

– What will set you free?

– What is your future?

– Do you have fun?

– Do you, have you?

– Do you stand for anything?

– Why do I hold myself back?

– What will it take, to take that next
  step?

– What are you learning?

– How fast are you?

– What will be the ending question?

– What would you like to express but
  can't?

– What would you write about?

– What have you watched over and over and over again?

– How do you start your day?

– How do you end your day?

– Do you do the same things every day and night?

– Have you ever written a love letter?

– Have you ever punched someone?

– Have you ever been ax throwing?

– Do you share everything on a first meet?

– Do you really care?

– Have you ever been at your worst and still loved yourself?

– Do you feel a part of a family?

- Do you tell yourself one more episode?

- How much more can you take/handle?

- What is design to you?

- What look do you try and go for?

- What is the most sought-after style?

- What do you claim to own?

- How many pictures are there?

- What am I to you?

- Who is your saving grace?

- Who have you passed up?

- One, two or three?

- What exceptions are you willing to make?

- Are you willing to behave?

- What are your desires?

- What pills are you on?

- Do you take vitamins?

- What were you doing in 2012?

- What does a star feel like?

- Why is there competition?

- Who really wants competition?

- Did you ever fall in love with something you were forced to do or pushed to be involved with?

- Do you stop and observe?

- Would you rather take things apart or put things back together?

- What is your mindset?

- What does mindset mean to you?

- Does the universe have a mind?

- What does your energy portray?

- Do you know you don't have to suffer all the time?

- What are you reminded of?

- How can I help?

- How do you use your hands to help?

- Does the universe have hands?

- Do God's hands really hold us sometimes?

- Where is your grace?

- How are you healing?

- How dark does it get before your dawn?

- Who do you have faith in?

- Do you believe in your way of life?

- Where is your light?

– Does anyone ever dust the ceilings?

– What is your favorite drink?

– Where is your favorite place to go?

– Who do you feel like hearing from?

– Why do animals return to their natural habitats?

– Why is change so hard?

– How does stress effect the body so much?

– Does stress effect the body more than anything else in the world?

– Can stress have a positive impact on the body, let alone in a person's life?

– Why do we refuse to change?

– What's the coldest place on the planet?

– What's the hottest thing on earth?

- What tree are you staring at?

- Can you look at yourself?

- What's behind you?

- Are you baffled?

- Where does hope lie?

- What are you doing?

- When asking someone how they are, do you really care?

- Does God want to know how we are doing?

- Chicken or beef?

- Watermelon or grapes?

- Tattoos or piercings?

- What car do you drive?

- Heat or cool?

- Under or over?

- Would you quit if it meant
  something better?

- Do you see things within things?

- What keeps you busy?

- How much have you paid attention
  to someone else's life?

- Could you live without electronics?

- Could you live without electricity?

- What is your power?

- How do you keep your fruit fresh?

- Did you go to prom?

- What is school like for you?

- Do you have true friends?

- What's your deadline?

- What gives you butterflies?

- What's breaking your wallet?

- How far is too far?

- Who are you worried about?

- What is your problem?

- New or old?

- How thoughtful are you?

- What are God's thoughts, does the universe know?

- Are you delusional?

- Who is really sane?

- Who are you willing to lose?

- Who have you lost?

- Who have you gained?

- Have you ever cheated?

- Have you been cheated on?

- Have you had to start over?

- Have you ever been to jail?

- What is your hell like?

- Is there such a thing as to many
  emotions?

- What do you want to hear?

- Would you give love another chance?

- Would you sell your most prized
  possession?

- Have you had your work in a gala?

- Do you like my dark side?

- Do you hurt the people you love?

- Why are things so bittersweet?

- How do you prefer to be?

– What's the best interview?

– What is the best?

– What are your habits?

– What is gone?

– What do you have hidden?

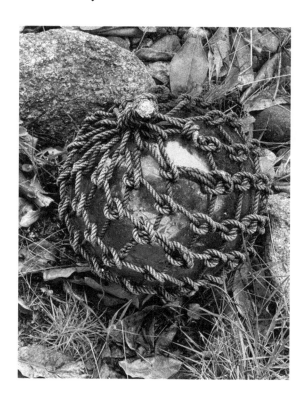

- How long does it take to get over someone?

- Why don't you answer?

- Do you really know who you are hanging out with?

- What's the best plan you've ever come up with?

- Have you been kicked out?

- What is your vision?

- What lines have been crossed?

- How many versions of the same story have been told differently?

- Have you been saved?

- Where have you flown to?

- Have you ever been on a ship?

- Have you ever been horseback riding?

- Can goals be endless?

- What is the perfect story?

- What do you have to lose by making your dreams come true?

- Do you have proof?

- Do you want to be done?

- Where to begin?

- Who would remember you after you're dead?

- What do you dread?

- What's the longest movie?

- Would you go down the rabbit hole?

- Are you happy for the ending?

- Can you temper everything about your life?

- Are you invited?

- Who came up with xoxo?

- Have you ever been on TV?

- What's one thing you've quit buying?

- How badly do you try to make new memories?

- How do you measure things?

- Are you tired?

- Should I let you know?

- Is it really written in stone?

- Has your story been written in the stars?

- What miracle would save you?

- Can you quake like a ....crazy person lol?

- Are you waking up?

- Who have you let down?

- What is a spiritual plain to you?

- What does forgiveness mean to you?

- Will I ever have a place to call my own or have I already had one?

- How do you remember what happened?

- What do you consider to be success?

- How many times have you broken up?

- How crazy can you get?

- What hair color do you prefer?

- What kind of wedding would you want?

- What amuses you?

- What is fancy to you?

- What is too soon to get married?

- Have you ever been locked in a room with no way out?

- What do you consider a healthy relationship?

- What feels right to you?

- Where do you find enjoyment?

- What promises have you broken?

- Have you accepted your past faults?

- Are you good at figuring things out?

- Does God eat?

- Is staying focused easier than we think it is?

- What's the best city to live it?

- If God does eat, what kinds of foods are preferred?

- Are you all packed?

– Who do you cry out to?

– Are you ignoring the signs?

– What are your needs?

– Why don't you reach out?

– What do you refuse to do?

– What are you talking about?

– What are your wishes?

– What's in your shoe box?

– What were your grades like?

– How do you consider yourself to be?

– Who are you when no one is around?

– Have you ever made any kind of
   donations?

– Would you look?

– Are you dating anyone?

– Have you left a mark in the world?

– What price would you pay?

– What chances are you taking?

– Where do you hang your heart?

– Are you glad you're not who you use to be?

– Who do you text the most?

– What's the shortest relationship you've been in?

– Do you know how to set boundaries?

– What happens at the end?

– What drama is in your life?

– What's the one thing you don't want to be real?

– Would you stay if it meant losing yourself in the process?

- Can you pick a lock?

- Can you see in the dark?

- Sharp or dull?

- Reading or writing?

- What side of the coin did you want?

- You wanted to be pricked by that rose didn't you, why else would you have played with It?

- How questionable is your character?

- What maze is your mind in?

- How do you wrap your mind around your thoughts?

- How soon will you be done?

- What music does your mind play?

- Does God play music and if so what kind?

- Is there pleasure in the rabbit hole that you seek?

- What makes you laugh?

- What are your dastardly thoughts in your mind?

- What keeps your eyes open at night?

- How do you feel about the universe?

- Have you ever been woken up by a storm?

- Is thunder God's way of making noise?

- Can you follow directions?

- Why can't I remember?

- Have you ever had to run for your life?

- Can you wait to get out of here?

- What new places have you tried lately?

- Do you realize people can see the faces you make?

- Can you sit in public and laugh out loud regardless of who's around you?

- What is one of your happiest moments?

- Can you blink your eyes and touch your nose at the same time?

- Did you, do it?

- Now why, why did you do it?

- Are you laughing? (Well, I am smiling hope you are!)

- Do you trust anyone?

- What are a few things in life that keep you going?

- Have you been struck by lightning?

- I wonder what it's like to be struck by lightning, do you?

- Where will your next escapade be?

- What are you doing to please someone else?

- If you went missing who would look for you?

- What anniversary do you celebrate?

- Where are you running off to?

- Do you write for yourself or others?

- What are you taking to the grave?

- What are you sorry for?

- What are your hopes?

- Did you ever feel apart from?

- Who's in love with you?

– Do you let negative words get in your way?

– What did you do wrong?

– What are you afraid to admit?

– What are your interests?

– What's unusual about your situation?

– Are you really living?

– What's been discovered lately?

– Are you staying safe?

– What has been taken from you?

– Do you receive messages that aren't meant for you

– Are you, someone else's fantasy?

– What ghosts haunt you?

– Do you leave notes?

- How many times have you had to practice something till you got it right?

- What conspiracies are you into?

- Who is saying what about you?

- Do you even care?

- What are you saying about who?

- Who is really innocent?

- What does guilty imply?

- What fun do you want to have today?

- What law would you get rid of?

- What law would you add?

- Why is there always war?

- Are you lucky?

- Do you believe your beautiful?

– What did I miss?

– Would you hurt you?

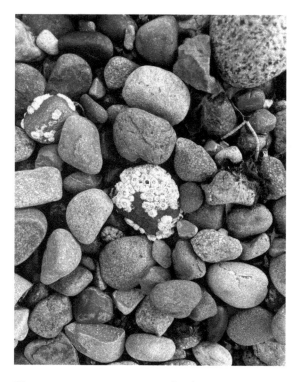

– Can you erase your feelings?

– Did you give into your emotions?

– What's making you overthink things?

- When did you meet up with a good friend last time?

- Are you worried about what others think?

- Would you tell someone else's secrets to save your own skin?

- What have you broken?

- Are you sassy?

- What's the last party that you've been to?

- Can time stand still?

- Has anyone come to your rescue?

- Have you been to another country?

- What colors don't go together?

- Have you gotten lost?

- Do you have a secret place?

- Did you mean to say that out loud?

- Are you there for people when they need you?

- Do you blow your mind?

- How many jobs do you have?

- How many careers do you have?

- Are any of these questions repeated in this book or in the last one?

- Have you finally had your chance?

- What looks different to you?

- How do you meet people?

- What's the longest power outage?

- Do you have things ready just in case there is an emergency?

- Do people understand you?

- Do you understand yourself?

– What is there to do in your town?

– Who is famous where you live?

– What are you most likely to do?

– How do you clean things?

– Are you going to be, okay?

– What's weird to you?

– Do you do social media of any kind?

– Do you watch the news?

– Has this been fun for you?

– What's been your favorite question so far?

– Where is it written that one must go on?

– What captures the best lighting?

– Where is the darkest place?

- Would you want a star named after you?

- Do you blare your music?

- Do you like to go to parties?

- What was one of the best parties ever thrown?

- Do you think you are doing good things?

- In who's eyes are you the villain?

- Are you someone's hero?

- What does it mean to be a hero?

- What does it mean to be a villain?

- What is sexuality to you?

- Is everything sexualized these days?

- What was the sexiest year?

- Have you bought your dream dress?

- Have you ever worn a crown?

- How easy is it to correct yourself?

- What is a tree to you?

- What does a tree feel like?

- What does cement feel like?

- What does the dirt feel like?

- How do your feet feel right now?

- How does your gut feel?

- Do you have a pet?

- Do you pay attention to shadows or light or both?

- Do you have a globe?

- How many books do you own?

- Do you think you're a mess?

- Do things need to be put better?

– What gives you goose bumps?

– Where is your next place to think going to be?

– Do you game for a living?

– Do you color and if so with what?

– How would you rather be?

– Do you like your family?

– Do you shave?

– Why does hair grow back?

– Why are things so expensive?

– Will I ever be able to support myself?

– Do you think you should write?

– Where are you sitting?

– Where is the place people stand the most?

- What God is sought after the most?

- Are the gods in any kind of competition?

- Are things really done by accident or by mistake if God really had them planned out that way in the first place?

- Where to go from here?

- What do you want to see in the world?

- What reflections do you desire?

- What does it mean to become what you respect?

- How do you mirror?

- Do you really want to get into this?

- Why not dating?

- What questions are you asked in a day, let alone in a week?

- Who do you tell to keep going it will get better?

- How far do you live?

- Are you bored?

- Can you find the time to do what you need to do?

- Where does time go?

- Why do things feel the way they do?

- Who came up with feelings?

- What's your point?

- Where is all of this coming from?

- Who came up with what?

- What's your lifelong dream?

- What's the longest goal you've set for yourself?

- Are we there yet?

- Here you go again why?

- What are you dragging your feet for?

- Will it get you?

- Why does it always burn?

- Where do corpuscles come from?

- Do you use auto text?

- Do you think you've gotten to know
  me through these questions?

- Do you think you've gotten to
  know yourself better through these
  questions?

- Do you think you gotten to know
  the world better through these
  questions?

- Are you glad you don't hang out with
  the people you used to?

- Did you feel that?

– What is the light that you seek?

– What did you bring in from yesterday?

– Are you back to your emotional self?

– Where do emotions go?

– Where are you hiding?

– Do you feel like you have wings at times?

– How do you stay connected?

– Who's standing on the outside of the groups you're in?

– Who thinks you're cool?

– Who wants to be a part of your life and is too afraid to step into it?

– Do you notice the outsiders anymore?

– Were you once an outsider?

- Did you or do you hang out with a mixture of people?

- Are you judgmental?

- What are your opinions?

- Do you have a favorite blanket you like to curl up with?

- Do you like to sit next to the fire?

- Is there truth in a lie and a lie in the truth?

- Are your eyes getting tired?

- Is it time for another cup of coffee or tea?

- What got you excited?

- Do you know that the people you know now you may not know or see later in life ever again?

- Are you enjoying the moment?

– Do you have stuffed animals?

– How many pillows do you have?

– Have you ever made a blanket?

– Have you realized yet that you can't really make others happy, you can barely make you happy?

– What is it about happiness that is so sought after?

– I need?

– I want?

– What are your weekend plans?

– What's got you upside down?

– Where are you going to be at after you accomplish your goals?

– Who checks up on you?

– Do you have a white rabbit?

– Did you become someone else
because of someone else?

– Who are you preforming for?

– Is your underwear drawer organized?

– Are you alone?

– What are you putting off?

– Where do you lay down to rest?

– Has anyone brought you flowers?

– Are you running out of things to
think about?

– How drunk are you?

– What's the most messed up that
you've been?

– Do you think people will wait for
you?

– Do you want to fall by the wayside?

– Did you know that everybody lies?

– How hard has it been?

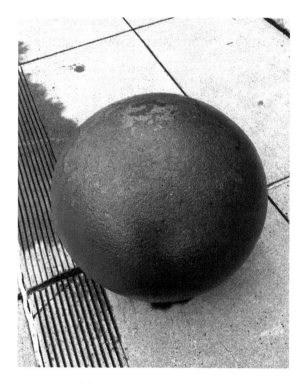

– Do you like how you sound when
you sing?

– Do you know how to play an
instrument?

- Do you have anyone to share with?

- I can't tell you it's a secret, how does that phrase affect you?

- Are we getting somewhere?

- What keeps you up at night?

- How do you wake up in the morning?

- Are you a risk taker?

- Do you talk to strangers?

- What does pink mean to you?

- What does purple mean to you?

- What do you think of when you hear the color orange?

- How were you the monster in someone else's fairytale?

- Have you been the monster in someone's life?

- Who's disturbing your peace?

- Who chained you up?

- What's made you sick?

- How clever are you?

- How far have you come from where you've been?

- Do you tell your kids things you shouldn't?

- What do you tell yourself to get through the day?

- What's real in your life?

- Do you have fake fruit?

- Where do you find your answers?

- How do you do your research?

- Who healed your broken heart?

- Do you use skin care?

- What are you a beginner at?

- Who do you say good morning to?

- Is a secret really a lie in disguise?

- Have you ever been rock climbing?

- Are you a thrill seeker?

- What is your favorite theme song?

- Do you have a favorite sweater?

- What are you sharing?

- What can you do?

- What are you willing to hear?

- What are you holding onto?

- Who are you into?

- How thick does the plot go?

- What did you miss?

– What's on top of your fridge?

– Have you been left behind?

– Have you ever been phony?

– Have you ever heard your child cry
and there wasn't anything you could
do?

– Can you disappear from social
media?

– What are you looking for?

– Can you stay put?

– Who said life was fair?

– What's your cliff hanger?

– Is saying no still hurtful?

– When will it be over?

– Are you ready for a new beginning?

– Does anyone make you food?

– Are you complicated?

– Who is your goat?

– Do you know how to belay?

– Do you know what belaying is?

– Have you belayed before?

– In going forward in your own
  happiness who have you left behind,
  have you noticed everyone that
  you've left.

– Do you listen to your heart?

– Who do you wish could come back?

– What do you see every day?

– Who would you lay next to?

– Black or white?

– Grey or beige?

– What name have you always wanted?

- Do you enjoy alone time?

- What choices should you be making?

- Are you a good wing man?

- What are feathers made of?

- What are you willing to do to help someone out?

- Have you had a therapy session?

- What do you guess?

- Is it up to you?

- What are you trying to stop?

- Where are you going?

- What does it take to get somewhere?

- What places should be traveled?

- Is your best friend also your worst enemy?

– What are you up to?

– Can you be open to other spiritual
  things?

– Do you check your bags?

– Do you believe love can come out of
  no where?

– How late can you stay up?

– What's the earliest you've gotten up?

– What's green?

– What's violet?

– What colors do you see?

– Can you be your own king?

– Who's yelling at you?

– Why do you shut out the world?

– How long have you been in the
  relationship that you're in?

– Are you trying to leave your mark on or in the world and if so, how?

– Can you see what they saw?

– Why is it considered suicide when they only want to take the pain away?

– What are your promises?

– Do you know what's in that building?

– What do you find delight in?

– What is joyful in your life?

– How big is your heart?

– What is your soul like?

– Where does smoke go?

– How are names made?

– Who are you waiting on to call you?

– Have you ended treatment?

- What changed?

- What are you saying?

- How old were you when you could remember your dreams?

- What's the longest vacation that you've ever taken?

- Have you ever acted like an animal?

- Where do you take yourself?

- What loops are you making?

- How many shades are there?

- Can someone get there sight back?

- Can you be trusted?

- How are you moving on?

- What scares you?

- Are you sorry?

– What's been difficult for you?

– What do you think of when you see a group of people or a big family?

– Have you ever worn a wig before?

– Who have you heard from lately?

– How do you feel when you haven't accomplished anything for a while?

– Can you take the high road?

– What's the rudest thing you've ever done?

– Are you finally getting back to where you need to be?

– Do dolls creep you out?

– Do you do what you're asked?

– Do you torture yourself?

– What are your memories?

- What do you think is not possible?

- Who would rescue you?

- Have you ever had a surprise kiss?

- What do you consider to be family?

- What's fun to you?

- What you wear, what does it say about you?

- How do people perceive you in the way you dress?

- Would you ask strangers about their opinion on the way you dress?

- How fast is a plane going when it touches the ground?

- What do you call a group of moose?

- Are you trying to escape life?

- What class do you consider yourself to be?

- What?

- Who did you meet?

- Would you want to get to know the people you're sitting next to?

- Will you ever meet again?

- Who would you donate to?

- What would you donate?

- How do you fly?

- How would you calm a friend down?

- What would you give up being there for someone else?

- Who?

- Where?

- When?

- Is now the right time?

– What do sound waves really do to the brain?

– Are your thoughts your friends?

– What love do yo have to give?

– Did you remember what you forgot?

– Have you ever done things on a whim?

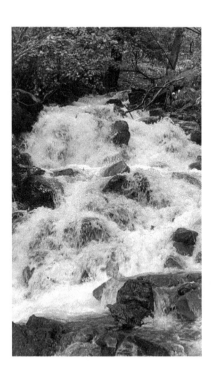

- Have you ever stayed with a complete stranger?

- Would you go get lost just for fun?

- Do you live in a place where someone died in that place, known or unknown?

- Does rain and crackling fire sound the same when slow?

- What are you trying to take from someone else?

- Have you read the signs?

- How close have you gotten?

- What don't you like?

- If no one deserves to die then, why do we all die?

- What have you solved?

- What is gone?

- What is liberty to you?

- How would you like to be remembered?

- What would you like to be remembered by or for?

- What's your favorite fruit?

- What adventure awaits you?

- Cats or dogs?

- What are you excited for?

- Can you ask nicely?

- What sounds are around you?

- Is the sun out?

- Can you tie a cherry stem in a knot?

- Do you have a scale?

- Do animals have patience?

– Have you mowed a lawn?

– Have you ever had to cut grass by hand?

– Why do farts stink so bad?

– Have you ever let your phone slowly die?

– What would you want to smell like?

– Who are you?

– What did you feel when the weather changed?

– How did you feel in a different state?

– What helps you relax?

– Do you like to snuggle?

– Have you ever seen a ghost?

– What kind of trouble have you been in?

- What's the longest you've watched TV for?

- What's bugging you?

- How do you connect with people?

- What traditions are you passing down?

- Have you a bonus in life?

- How do you see things?

- Who do you write about?

- What is going on in your mind?

- What are your plans for this week?

- Have you been forgotten?

- What fears are holding you back?

- What do you like to eat?

- Have you ever let your makeup run while the tears fell?

- Have you ever reapplied your makeup after crying?

- Have you ever been to a gay bar?

- Would you meet with your enemy?

- Have you ever been followed?

- Have you ever followed someone?

- What do you do on your rainy days?

- Would you rather cuddle with a person or an animal?

- Have you ever had to sign a DNR?

- What does time mean to you?

- What are you looking for?

- What are you throwing away?

- How much space do you need?

- Why is it hard to go back?

– What flowers do you like?

– Who was there for you growing up?

– Are you longing for human connection?

– Did you know dogs eat toenails?

– Did everything check out?

– How do you help?

– Are you really happy?

– What's changing in your life?

– How many things are made of glass?

– What works under water?

– Who's a stranger in your life?

– Would animals tell our secrets if they could talk?

– What do you keep in your pockets?

- What do like to look at?

- What do you meditate on the most?

- Have you ever made a dream catcher?

- What have you made lately?

- What hidden talents do you have?

- Would you write down all your secrets if it meant no one else would or could see them?

- Have you asked someone lately what they would like to do?

- Have you asked anyone what they would want?

- Are you happy with the people in your life?

- Do you have a hard time meeting new people?

- How well are you?

- Where do you get most of your work done?

- What kind of work do you do?

- Do you like the sound of silence?

- What's that sound?

- What do you have on display that you don't even use?

- What would you do if you got called out onto the ledge?

- What battles are you choosing to fight?

- Have you ever seen someone attempting suicide on the side of a building ten stories high?

- Are you standing where somebody jumped?

- What's your white rabbit and where is the hole you're willing to go down?

– Who would you travel to go see?

– Would you still complain if there was no one around?

– Do you get privacy?

– Have you ever been in a race?

– What is your rush?

– What is inner peace to you?

– How do you get things accomplished?

– How excited are you?

– Are you sad?

– Have you ever had all your emotions hit you all at once and if so, what were they?

– Have you listened to any new music lately?

- What new places have you checked out?

- What nerves have you tried?

- What are you eating?

- When's the last time you thought for you?

- What's the last thing you kissed?

- Have you walked in the rain?

- What do you appreciate?

- How hard do you work?

- Do you like who you work with?

- Do you like or even know who you're surrounded by?

- What is free anymore?

- Do you feel welcomed?

- What have you said goodbye to?

- What do you stand for?

- Will you finish in time?

- What don't you want to be doing anymore?

- Is food another form of a drug?

- What are you willing to try?

- What is attractive to you?

- What hurt you?

- Are you staying warm?

- Do you have someone you can count on?

- Do you like what you hear?

- What history do you know?

- What do you know about the present moment?

- What are you drinking?

- What are you teaching others around you?

- What's okay to you?

- What do you buy too much of?

- What colors do you see?

- Do you feel threatened?

- What questions don't you like?

- What's crazy to you?

- What's your favorite question?

- Do you trust technology? Why or why not?

- Is what is in one state in another state?

- Do you want to keep to yourself?

- What are you developing?

- Are you staying clean?

– Why do you buy books?

– What jokes do you tell?

– Do you find humor in sorrow?

– What kind of music do you like?

– Have you ever colored with crayons as an adult?

– Do you color inside the lines?

– Do you respect the crazy ones?

– Have you ever gone crazy?

– When was your first suicidal thoughts and why?

– Can you quit buying things?

– Are you waiting on the weather?

– Are you tired?

– What is your energy level at?

- Do you care if others hear your conversation?

- How long have you been gone for?

- Where does your heart lead you?

- What does your head tell you?

- What does your hell say about you?

- Have you ever seen someone break down and cry?

- Can you find happy?

- What color is happy?

- What is pink?

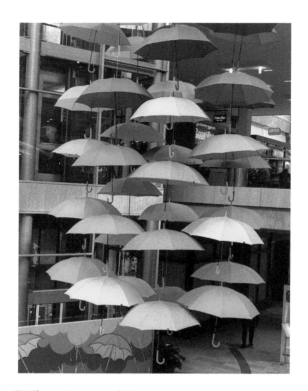

- What is peach?

- What is brown?

- What color is caring?

- What color is hatred?

- What color is love?

— Where do you define your colors in your life?

— What did you accidentally throw away?

— What helps you remember things?

— Is there a place you'd rather be?

— Have you ever had to dig in the trash?

— Have you ever been in a hammock?

— What's the worst itch that you've ever had?

— What's the worst thing you've been through?

— What's the best thing you've been through?

— Are you waiting on something in the mail?

— Do you ever observe people?

- What are your desires?

- Who are you looking for?

- What's silly in your life?

- Do you like the atmosphere?

- Do you like the attention that you're getting?

- What makes you nervous?

- What sweet smells are around you?

- Have you given anyone a compliment lately?

- Why are you staying put?

- Who have you said hi to lately?

- What do you like to take photos of?

- Are you stuck?

- Who do you inspire?

- Who interests you?

- What holiday do you like?

- What frightens you?

- Who would you want to play?

- Who do you want to believe in you?

- What do you want to stop?

- What costumes would you wear?

- Have you gotten used to the sounds around you?

- Do you think it's warm when the sun is out?

- What's the longest you've been on hold?

- Has your bravery changed over your lifetime?

- Have you figured out the way yet?

- Do you remember the Macarena?

- What were you doing on 9/11?

- When's the last time you got injured?

- What do you believe will hold you up?

- What friends have you made lately?

- What's your next destination?

- Who was your childhood crush?

- Have you ever had a tooth ache?

- Do you know what it's like to hav a prosthetic?

- What's the weather like?

- What is fresh air?

- Is there any where you want to be taken to?

- What are you ready for?

– What are you starting?

– Where have you walked to?

– What pictures have you taken lately?

– Do you care about other people?

– Would you serve?

– What flags would you fly?

– What does your walk say about you?

– Is there anything else that you want to do?

– Are you in your dream job?

– What have you mended?

– Do you like art?

– Is the fire your friend?

– What did you have for breakfast?

– Who did you text last?

– Who was your last kiss?

– Are you enjoying you?

– What else is there to do?

– If you were to make a restaurant,
  what would it be and where would it
  be?

– What are you concerned about?

– Do questions change, like answers?

– What's your story?

– What do people say about you, do
  you know?

– What's the same?

– What does your heartbeat sound
  like?

– Do you leave messages?

– What is tracked?

- What is copied?

- How many things are copied?

- Are you copied?

- How many new numbers have you had?

- What made you change your number?

- Will you keep this number longer this time?

- Do you like to walk in the rain?

- Have you been mistaken for someone else?

- How busy is too busy?

- What gets you all antsy?

- What gives you goosebumps?

- Is your soul empty or full?

- What belongs to you?

- Have you ever lost control of anything including yourself?

- Do you love a simple life?

- What's locked down?

- Where are you coming from?

- Why do we all eat at the same time?

- Can one person be left alone their entire life and be, ok?

- Who's helping you out?

- I think it's time to leave do you?

- Do you have answers to things that don't exist?

- What do you eat?

- Can an answer even be looked up before a question is even read?

– What's everyday look like to you?

– Who calls you?

– Do you notice who comes and goes?

– Do you see the hidden message/
messages?

– Are you okay with making mistakes?

– Do you like fresh air?

– Do you like the sound of an engine
revving?

– Have you ever worked on a car or
motorcycle?

– Have you ever felt your body
buzzing?

– Have you ever felt shaky?

– What's it like to be healthy?

– Have you had to work hard for
everything you have?

– Can silence or noise kill someone?

– Is silence or noise inspiring and if so, which one is more inspirational?

– Are you cold?

– What temperature is your favorite?

– What's stoping you from doing what you want?

– Would you get a face tattoo?

– What are you doing today?

– What is the elevation where you are at?

– Where were you born?

– Who do you live with?

– What's got you on edge?

– Do you wish the end was near?

– Is the end near?

- Have you enjoyed some of your experiences?

- What's some of your most favorite experiences that you've had?

- Would you have done what you do without the support that you have? Or don't have?

- Have you ever walked somewhere to find out they were closed?

- Are you okay with the company you keep?

- Are you on time?

- Do you think that all colors are pretty?

- Are you surprised?

- Is anything negotiable in your life?

- Do you act as if?

- How did angel wings come about?

- How does your truth affect others?

- What is tough for you?

- What have you seen?

- What words bother you?

- What are some of your favorite words?

- What words can't you say?

- If something can't be imagined, can it still be created?

- Do you hear the silent whispers?

- What are you living for?

- What is love to you?

- Have you been in a helicopter?

- What is your legacy?

- Have you danced under the disco ball?

– How far have you taken yourself?

– How many lives are saved?

– How many times has your life been saved?

– Can meditation consist of seeing how others are doing?

– What does your first cup of coffee do for you?

– How much more do you have left before you are finished?

– Do you take you out on dates?

– What gives you the feel good bumps?

– Where do you like to work?

– What kind of art do you like to look at?

– What did you eat last?

– Are you a patient?

- How many people do you see?

- How many things can you see?

- What catches your attention the most?

- What do you pour your heart out to/ into?

- What do you consider to be fair?

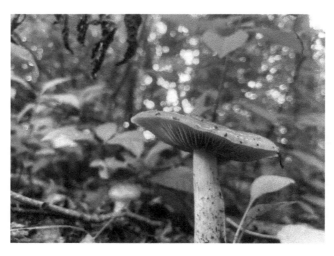

- What do you want to learn about and why haven't you learned about it yet?

- Do you like fall?

– How do you feel about pumpkins?

– How does a pumpkin feel?

– Has your name been called?

– How does rain feel?

– What is snow to you?

– What is your ideal climate?

– Are you forgiving?

– What do you honor?

– Do you have respect for anyone or even for yourself?

– Do you have trust issues?

– Does anyone remind you of anyone?

– Have you ever taken a picture of a stranger?

– Have you ever asked a stranger to take a picture?

- What are your excuses?

- What kind of day do you work best on?

- What chances are you taking?

- Do you get excited for a text?

- Have you ever used a land line?

- What do you do so you can go on vacation?

- Do you reach out to people only if you need something?

- Who are you looking for?

- Would someone offer a reward to find you?

- What does life mean to you?

- Is there a cure all?

- Are you still dreaming?

- What did you dream about last night?

- Have you set a goal in a while?

- Do you know what it really means to believe in something or someone?

- How do you try and simplify your life?

- Why is gum like slime?

- Do you know how tall you are?

- What is your eye color?

- How sick are you?

- Have you ever mapped out where you were going?

- How many names do you go by?

- Can you handle grief?

- Are you emotional?

- Do you know what triggers your emotions?

- What's your way of disconnecting?

- Do you believe in prayer?

- Do you believe in mercy?

- What is mercy to you?

- What answer are you getting?

- What cycles are happening in your life?

- Can you save yourself?

- What would you do if you got a tail?

- Does your fire burn bright?

- Can you feel anything?

- Have you had to leave a life behind?

- Have you ever had to choose one life over the other?

– How silly are you?

– What is strange about you?

– Do animals see spirits?

– Do you want to learn the truth?

– Are you going to new places?

– Do you like routine?

– What is it about change that people don't like?

– What are love birds to you?

– Does art inspire you?

– What animal speaks to you the most?

– Can you turn down a gift?

– What gifts do you give?

– Why are wolves considered to be tricksters?

- Have you ever howled with the wolves?

- What sparks your thoughts?

- What do designs inspire in people?

- Have you signed your life away?

- Has your life begun?

- Are you willing to go to any lengths to have a better life?

- Are you staring cause you like what you're looking at?

- Why does it feel like I've done this before even though I haven't?

- How do you like your bacon?

- What are you good at remembering?

- Do you enjoy what you eat?

- When your head goes down, where do your feet go?

– What are you done hearing about?

– What color do you need more of in your life?

– Do you play with numbers and letters?

– Have you helped someone take a photo?

– What's your flight like?

– Do you understand other people?

– What clouds are there?

– Have you eaten?

– What's the highest elevation that you've ever been?

– What's too bright for you?

– Can you duck and cover?

– What's too dark for you?

- What are you trying to quit in your life?

- Where is your space at?

- Have you leveled out yet?

- Do you like daylight?

- What if the things we thought were fake were real and the things that were real were fake?

- Can you fly?

- Where have you flown to?

- What fears have you overcome?

- Are you indulging in things that you shouldn't?

- What limits have been placed on you?

- Can you fall asleep easily?

- Can you sleep anywhere?

- Does turbulence scare you?

- What's the longest flight you've been on?

- How kind are you?

- Do you like to talk with people?

- What music inspires you?

- Do you take adventures?

- Where are we going today?

- What's blinding you from seeing the truth?

- What's hurting you the most right now?

- Who are you missing?

- Could you do a staycation?

- What if anything can you say has inspired you?

- Do you like clouds?

- What weather is your favorite?

- Do you fidget?

- Can you see what's in front of you?

- Have you ever blindly texted?

- Have you ever written in the dark then read it the next day, and was it readable?

- Who are you calling out to?

- Who do you not know in your family?

- Do you wear ear buds or headphones?

- What do you drink?

- What makes you lightheaded?

- Have you blown kisses to heaven or hell?

– What's the sleepiest that you've ever been?

– Do you wear jewelry?

– Does the sunshine brighten your life?

– Have you ever flown by yourself before?

– Who farted?

– Have you ever been stuck somewhere with a bad smell?

– Have you seen the endless beauty of life and death?

– Did you mind getting distracted?

– Why do some clouds look like waves?

– How were cotton balls discovered and how are they made?

– Are you tired yet?

– What do you wish would happen?

– What might be better for you?

– Can you hear your own crazy?

– What do you think you don't deserve?

– What sounds are beautiful to you?

– Would you step inside your mind let alone your soul given the chance?

– What traces have you left?

– What are you denying yourself?

– What freedoms have been taken away from you?

– Do you like trouble?

– What's more important to you being right or being at peace?

– How does it feel to be turned sideways to you?

– Are you a shape you want to be?

– Are you who you want to be?

– What's it going to take for you to feel accomplished let alone accepted?

– Do pilots ever get bored during a flight?

– Have pilots gotten lost or still get lost sometimes?

– Have you ever lost your luggage?

– Has your luggage ever been lost?

– What's the best way to travel?

– Who understands you?

– How well do you travel?

– How low can you go?

– Have you ever walked on hot coals?

– Would you ever go glacier rafting?

– Would you go rock climbing?

– What are you sweeping under the rug?

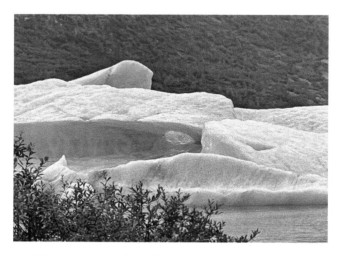

– How many hidden objects are there?

– What have you discovered lately?

– Are you okay with rescheduling?

– What are you willing to try?

– How much longer?

– What word combinations shouldn't be put together?

- Do you notice what the universe is trying to tell you?

- Are you brave?

- Why are there tiny wholes in airplane windows?

- What picture have you captured on a plane?

- What notes do you take?

- Who would you sit next to given a chance?

- Do you follow the rules?

- Has an airplane ever run out of gas while taxiing?

- Why is oxygen running out?

- Why do we think we know the answers?

- What are you proud of?

- What things do you like to do?

- Have you ever cut a trip short?

- Have you ever been chased by a
  bear?

- If you had a chance to save a life,
  who's life would you save?

- Have you ever taken a photo with the
  firemen?

- Who do you look like?

- Can you accept things as they are?

- Why do clouds look like to angels?

- Can angels sit on clouds?

- What should we do today?

- Have you ever gone to a stranger's
  graveside?

- Where do you want your resting
  place to be?

– Do trees ever get cold?

– What are you excited about today?

– What changed your mind?

– Who have you been thankful for?

– Do you hear the little animals?

– Can you hear the noise of the city and the silence of your mind?

– Have you blown smoke away?

– Have you ever closed your eyes and listened to your surroundings?

– Have you ever sat in seven minutes of silence?

– What defense skills do you know?

– Are you someone's distraction?

– Do you like to hang out or do you have other intentions?

- Do you use lighters or matches?

- Do you walk barefoot?

- What waters have you put your feet into?

- Have you ever walked on sacred ground?

- Have some of your allergies gone away?

- What animals have you learned about?

- What new sounds have you heard lately?

- What's making that sound?

- How do you feel about hiccups?

- What's on your to do list?

- Do you like the sounds of nature?

- Have you ever sat so silently that nature was so loud you forgot where you were?

- You ever hear something that sounded closer than it really was?

- How many little animals are there?

- What kind of services have you been to?

- How many churches have you been to?

- How many gravesides have you visited?

- How do you drink your coffee?

- How do you eat your strawberries?

- What do you have for breakfast?

- How do you like to start your week?

- What do you ask God?

- Does the universe help you?

- Do you help the universe?

- What do you give back in order to be helpful?

- Why do certain animals sound like they are screaming?

- Do you like the smell of smoke?

- What colors do you like in the leaves?

- Crows or ravens?

- Squirrels or chipmunks?

- What are you thinking?

- How do you learn about things about the universe in the universe?

- Are you okay with not correcting someone or yourself?

- How late did you stay up?

- What was the last argument you had about?

- How do you respond when someone is trying to argue with you?

- What do you do when someone tries to be aggressive towards you?

- Do you cry to stop from yelling?

- How do you handle public humiliation?

- Can you accept someone else getting all the attention?

- If you get miss treated, do you take it out on others or on yourself?

- What was the best part about your day?

- It's not okay to be miss treated, is it?

- When is enough, enough?

– Can you stop before your breaking point?

– Where do you draw the line and why are you drawing it?

– Why do you have buttons to be pushed?

– Do you take deep breaths to refresh the mind and the body?

– How do you reset yourself throughout the day?

– What is your go to activity that keeps you going?

– What do you work on in the middle of the night?

– Do you think you ever have peace?

– When do you get the most peace in your day?

– Wow who thought Washington would be quieter than Alaska?

– Have you ever heard a pin drop?

– Is there hope for humanity?

– How well can you hear?

– How well can you see?

– Do you appreciate your senses?

– Do you know what your senses are?

– How well do you communicate?

– Do you assume a lot, and does it get you into trouble?

– How early is too early?

– Did you know that I was up with you at that time?

– Do you believe in coincidence or that things happen for a reason?

– Do you believe in magic?

- How do you feel about manifesting things into reality?

- What are your thoughts on some people being linked together in one way or another?

- How close are you to the people you know?

- What is it that attracts you to the things you do every day?

- Do you ever hide in the dark?

- Can you see in the dark?

- What do you allow in your life?

- Have you ever been to the bigger cities?

- Have you ever hiked Mt. Rainier?

- What other things in this lifetime do you want to do?

- What breaks your peace?

- What gets you jumpy? (noises, places, people, etc.)

- What animal do you relate to the most?

- Are you ever carefree?

- What is it about black that freaks most people out?

- Do you enjoy what you are working on?

- Would you walk in someone else's shoes given the chance?

- Would you fly with the birds?

- Have you swum with the dolphins?

- Would you swim with the sharks?

- Do you want to swim with the turtles?

- What islands would you like to visit?

- What do tattoos represent to you?

- Have you gotten an out of state tattoo?

- Where do you go for the winter?

- What's the best thing you've ever tasted?

- What's the worst thing you've ever tasted?

- Is your head in the clouds?

- Do you know how you deserve to be treated?

- How well do you know the different animals in your area?

- Have you ever been called stuck up?

- Do you care how your hair looks?

- Are you okay with playing games with different rules or not by the rules at all?

- What rules do you follow?

- Can you color outside the lines?

- What's in your pot?

- Do you know how to cook?

- Do you stay up all day?

- Have you helped anyone today?

- What's it like to be in total darkness?

- Do you wait for an answer after you
  ask a question?

- Can you tell the difference between
  the sounds of a squirrel and a bird?

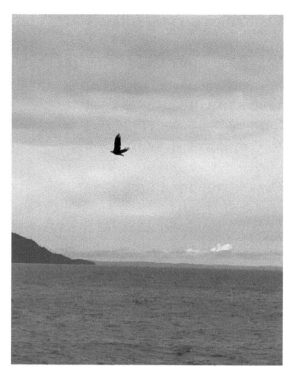

– Are you there for the ones you care about?

– Do you show moral support if asked to?

– What is emptiness?

– Where do you begin to change?

- Do you believe in numerology?

- Do you believe we are connected to the universe?

- Are you enjoying what the universe has to offer you?

- Do you walk barefoot?

- Have you ever planted a tree?

- Have you ever planted a garden?

- Are you happy with all the tattoos you have gotten?

- Are you done getting tattooed yet?

- What do you find pleasure in?

- Blinds or curtains?

- Bunnies or birds?

- Grass or gravel?

- House or apartment?

- How big would you want your home to be?

- What are your excuses?

- How do you like to read a book?

- Courage or strength?

- Do you chew on things like gum?

- Have you ever been a pet sitter?

- What's your ideal job?

- Is sunbathing another form of meditation?

- How much do you got going on?

- How many things do you have playing all at once?

- Are you overwhelmed?

- Does to much noise make you nauseous?

- Who do you ask for a ride from?

- Did you enjoy getting a face tattoo?

- Would you ever consider getting permanent makeup done?

- Have you ever gotten a business loan before?

- Have you had your own company?

- What's stopping you from taking that action to a different lifestyle choice?

- Are you good at cooking?

- Have you ever been on a sinking ship?

- What is your makeup regimen like?

- Do you like your feet?

- Can you roll your eyes?

- Can you roll your tongue?

- Can you purr like a kitten?

- Do you appreciate you?

- Do you make lists?

- What are you grateful for?

- Have you ever been in an accident? If so what kind?

- Pen or pencil?

- How many doors are there?

- Do you know what an apostate is?

- What is a window to you?

- How do you define a definition?

- How many lamps are there?

- What kind of light bulb do you use?

- How many types of light bulbs are there?

– What's in your closet?

– Do you even have a closet?

– What do you say behind closed doors?

– Do you keep tally on things?

– Are you chasing the white rabbit?

– What is your zodiac sign?

– Did you know that there are really thirteen zodiac signs?

– Now what's your real zodiac sign?

– Did that mess you up?

– When you're sorry are you?

– Do you like shadows?

– Have you ever done shadow puppets?

– How many kinds of puppets are there?

- How do you wake up?

- Have you ever tried to count the stars?

- Have you ever attempted to count your hair strands?

- What is your favorite smell in the morning?

- What is your favorite smell throughout the day?

- What smell do you prefer at nighttime?

- Aaaw silence do you like it?

- Do you leave the TV on but keep the volume off?

- Do you like cartoons?

- Are you stuck in the past?

- Will you ever move forward?

- What breaks you of your habits?

- What's too much?

- What's not enough?

- Where do all the roots go?

- Have you ever eaten fresh off the vine street fruit?

- How early is too early?

- What do you listen to?

- Who do you invite into your life?

- What continues circles are in your life?

- What words can you not find?

- Are you speechless yet?

- What is clear?

- What is white?

- What is tan?

- How many different bird noises are there and what do they sound like?

- Have you heard every bird on the planet?

- What animals have you heard?

- What animals do you want to hear?

- What have you studied?

- Are you going to school for what you truly want or are you going for someone else?

- Did or do you have a favorite teacher?

- Why do we forget so easily?

- How much information can the brain store?

- Do we remember everything even if we can't recall what everything is?

- Dress or skirt?

- Pants or shorts?

- Shirt or tank top?

- Boots or sandals?

- How many new words are created every year?

- Why do we change words throughout time?

- What's that bird out the window, is it a stellar jay?

- What states have you been to?

- Have you ever made a funny face before?

- Can you raise one eyebrow and smile at the same time?

- Did you just try it?

- Did you look in the mirror and do it?

– Are you laughing yet?

– Now you can say you've made a funny face, can't you?

– Are you smiling yet?

– Can you whistle?

– Can you chew gum and talk at the same time?

– Is there anything you can't do?

– What have you done for yourself lately?

– Do you feel accomplished?

– How many shoes do you own?

– How many hoodies do you have?

– What are somethings you could give away?

– Have you ever had a yard sale?

– Have you ever had a moving sale?

– What's it like to move from another country?

– What do you imagine about?

– What's art to you?

– What's music to you?

– What's the world to you?

– What does standing your ground mean to you?

– Are you willing to take charge if you had to?

– How much time do you need to get ready for the day?

– Do you wear perfume or other smells?

– What's your hair type?

– What's your skin type?

- Do you know what time to leave to get where you need to be?

- How many different kinds of transportation are there?

- How many kinds of transactions are there?

- How many different kinds of currency are there?

- Have you been to another country?

- What country do you want to go to?

- What research have you done lately?

- Have you ever felt chest pains before?

- Do you want to go somewhere warmer for the winter?

- What are you too busy doing to be living?

- Who are you loving today?

- Is the air clean where you are?

- Have you burned a candle lately?

- When's the last time you watched a flame and lost track of time?

- Purse or backpack?

- Have you done everything you can?

- Who's your peanut gallery?

- What's got your tummy rumbling?

- Do you wish you could do more?

- Do you feel satisfied?

- What is your dying wish?

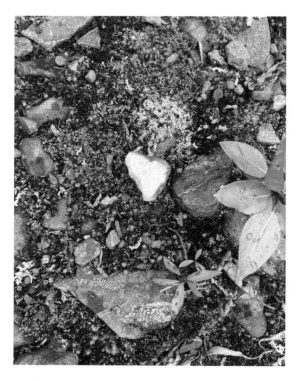

- Who do you want to see happy

- Who would you donate money to for
a good cause?

- Would you donate your time?

- How many things get donated?

- Do you appreciate what you have in your life?

- What's going on in your life?

- Do you understand the symbology behind what you collect?

- Is God even listening?

- How do you know God even hears you?

- Are you sick of the noise yet?

- What do you miss?

- Where do things go over time?

- What tragedy just happened?

- Why are there so many sirens?

- How many cop cars are there?

- Do all emergency vehicles get used?

- What sound do you find annoying?

- Do you have future plans and why not do them now?

- Can you keep going like you are?

- Have you ever slept a day away?

- Have you ever had anyone come check up on you?

- Have you found out the problem yet?

- Do you want to go to space?

- Are your thoughts your thoughts?

- How many dimensions are there?

- Would you offer yourself to save another?

- What are you fighting?

- Can you be willing?

- Do you have any marbles?

- Have you seen how a marble is made?

- Do you know how bricks are made? (by hand and the other way?)

- Have you seen candy being made?

- Have you ever made a candle?

- Do you know how to make candy?

- Do you know how electricity works?

- Have you built a fire?

- Have you ever locked yourself out of your house and or your car?

- What's your favorite show to watch?

- Far or near?

- Can getting lost be a form of meditation?

- Do you always look for answers in the same places?

– Are you covered?

– What have your choices brought you/ led up to?

– Do you like the sunshine on your face?

– Have you ever hung upside down for a different perspective?

– What keeps turning and stops abruptly?

– What keeps moving forward and eventually comes to an end?

– Eye spy with my little eye?

– What games did you play as a kid?

– Do you play any games now, what ones?

– What will you be for Halloween?

– Have you ever died your hair?

– Have you ever straightened your hair?

– Have you ever curled your hair?

– What have you done to your hair?

– What changes have you made to your body?

– What changes have happened to your body?

– What sits still and only moves to see?

– What only moves up and down?

– What is completely stationary?

– Does the wind make you cold?

– What's changing in your life?

– What changes and always moves directions?

– What can go through anything without showing any emotions?

- What color are your nails?

- What color are your lips?

- What do you put out to the universe?

- What does the breeze feel like?

- How hard does the wind blow?

- Are you excited for your next adventure?

- Do you help people when they fall down?

- What do you watch on TV?

- How many pages were in my last book?

- What are you stressed about?

- Who do you call baby?

- What things have you done that you've wanted to do?

– Are we in a spiritual crazy time?

– What made you cry last time?

– How do I look to you?

– Would you write me a letter?

– What would it say?

– Where is your key to your happiness?

– Why is it that we look outward for peace?

– If the water isn't safe to play in, then how is it the fish are safe to eat?

– Is anyone not wounded?

– Is anything sacred anymore?

– Can you hear the wind?

– How many stairs can you climb?

– What's the worst storm you've been in?

- How much do you weigh?

- What weight can you carry out?

- How hot can you handle?

- How cold can you handle?

- Have you ever looked for gold?

- What does letting go mean to you?

- What are you always thinking about?

- What do you always do every day?

- Would you chase a storm?

- Can you see where you're going?

- Are you a doomsday prepared?

- Are you afraid of the future?

- Do you live for today?

- What is your weapon in life?

– What is your choice?

– Where do you strive the most?

– What bugs you?

– Are you safe with what you do?

– What patterns do you like?

– How many street numbers are there?

– Do you know what you support?

– Did you ever think you'd make it big?

– What patterns in life do you always end up doing, that you try to break?

– What do you live for?

– Are you a hostage to your past?

– Have you ever eaten breakfast outside while the sun is shining, and a thunderstorm is rolling in?

– Do you scratch what itches?

– Have you roasted marshmallows?

– Are you leaving?

– What are you sipping on?

– Have you ever had to escape?

– What's made you feel scared?

– What do you pack around with you?

– What's the main thing you drink?

– What are your medical problems?

– Do you eat healthy?

– What is it about goals that when
  finished makes us feel better?

– How many questions will end up
  being in this book?

– Are you okay today?

- Are you afraid of spiders?

- Do you kill things?

- How do you enjoy life?

- What changes are you using in your life?

- Does music help you think?

- Can you find your way back?

- Do you reach out to strangers?

- Have you ever given your number to a random person?

- How cold are you?

- Rainbows or roses?

- What's the longest you've gone without a shower?

- Is it time to play yet?

- How many viruses are out there?

– How many infections are there?

– How many surgeries have you had?

– Are you ready for change?

– Are you the master of your life?

– Do you see that you are beautiful?

– What are your spirit animals?

– How many different kinds of tea is there?

– Have you ever tried juniper tea?

– Do you have any siblings?

– Can you draw?

– Have you walked a mile in someone else's shoes?

– Will war ever end?

– Would you change your career at the last minute?

– What demons have you created?

– What does it mean to be at peace?

– Who is the most relaxing person to be around?

– How many cats are there?

– How many dogs are there?

– What place is the least visited?

– Have you ever been on a sand dune?

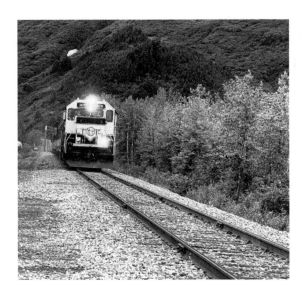

– Have you ever touched a glacier?

– How would you parent?

– What's the one thing you want most in the world?

– Can one really let go of their ego?

– What do you see when you look in the mirror?

– What do you consider to be family?

– What kind of beat gets you to want to dance?

– Do you know how to dance?

– Are you excited to get home?

– Are there people missing you?

– Are you ever really alone?

– What does ego mean to you?

– Where do you stand for solitude?

– How do you do your laundry?

– How much luggage do you pack when going on a trip?

– When will be the next trip?

– Where will be the next trip?

– Are you ready for whatever is coming next?

– What is it about the unknown that freaks out some and interests others?

– What is black but full of color?

– What stands still but always gets used?

– Are you okay with sudden moves?

– Are you okay with loud noises?

– What is the most moved thing?

– How much laundry is done in a day?

- What's the oldest thing you have?

- What do you consider to be old?

- What is young to you?

- What is considered a party?

- What is covered but you can see through?

- Are you distracted?

- Are you distributed?

- Do you understand the words in which you speak?

- How many words are written in a day?

- Is white really the absence of all colors, if so, then why is it needed to help create colors?

- What trust issues do you have?

- What makes us forget?

– Can you take it slow?

– Have you been abused?

– What are your warning signs?

– Would you take my hand for help?

– What are you a sucker for?

– What do you rebel against?

– Are you giving up?

– Are you loyal?

– Do you talk to yourself?

– How many questions have you not answered yet?

– Have you ever been stung by a bee?

– What are you allergic to?

– What smells good but tastes gross?

– What smells gross but tastes good?

- What do you beg for?

- Have you ever found a four-leaf clover?

- Do you wear jewelry?

- How do you listen to your music?

- What's always making noise but never moves?

- Do you think that you're courageous?

- What knocks you down?

- What do you sing?

- Do you see signs from angels?

- Do you know what it means to be alone?

- What do you worry about?

- What are you nearby?

– What's coming to an end?

– What makes you cry?

– Can you say I love you to another person and mean it ever again?

– Will the pain of loss ever go away?

– Why do we lie to ourselves?

– Did you mean to make me cry?

– Have you learned to laugh again?

– Are you smiling in the spirit world?

– Why do we torture ourselves?

– Does crying really cleanse the soul?

– Do you get your life together?

– When traveling, do you have set plans?

– Have you ever been arrested?

- Have you ever been in jail?

- Do you know it's okay to make mistakes?

- What's your proof?

- Where do you place the blame?

- Are you able to solve your problems?

- Do you pray for help?

- Do you ask for forgiveness?

- Where do you put your love towards?

- Can you get what you want accomplished soon?

- Do you use GPS?

- What kind of pictures do you take?

- Have you cried with anyone?

- What's the last movie you watched?

- Are you good at following through with what you say you're going to do?

- What do you think about yourself?

- What's one tattoo you wouldn't ever get?

- What's a piercing you wouldn't get?

- What have you been tested for?

- Have you split wood before?

- When's the last time you were by a fire?

- Can you relax?

- What are you anxious about?

- Are you good at waiting?

- What truth do you know?

- Are you relaxed yet?

– Do you answer a question with a question?

– Do you react or act when in a situation?

– What kind of struggles have you been through lately?

– How deep can you get?

– What is sex to you?

– When did you learn about sex?

– Do you like to learn new things?

– How far have you come?

– How many different colors do leaves change?

– What dies and can come back to life?

– Have you ever had a near death experience?

– What was your last thing you did?

- How many hats do you own?

- How long can you go without buying anything?

- Can you handle your emotions?

- What emotions are you feeling now?

- Can people count on you?

- What is your best quality?

- Where would you migrate to if you could?

- What's the most excited you've been and what was it over?

- When's the last time you got flowers?

- Have you ever bought flowers for yourself?

- Do you celebrate angel anniversaries?

- Are you able to do all the things you want to?

- What's your favorite time of year?

- How many bags do you own?

- Do you need to downsize?

- Is it time to have a yard sale or an art sale?

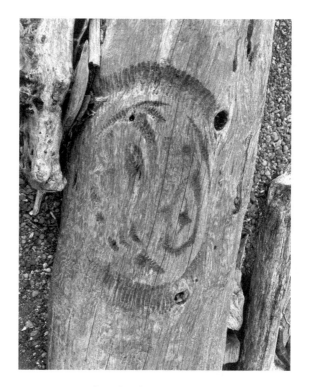

- How much cloths do you have?

– Are you willing to downsize or let go of some of your things?

– What time is it?

– Where does you story begin?

– How many friends do you have?

– How many family members do you really know?

– Do you know your family history?

– Who do you wish well to?

– Are you going to stay up all night?

– What does writing do for you?

– How do you escape life?

– What has an answer with no question?

– Do you like where you sleep?

– Are you comfortable?

– What would help you become a
  better person?

– Have you ever had a massage?

– Have you been to a hot spring?

– Have you been in a hot tub?

– Have you left a message in a bottle?

– Have you been to the ocean?

– Do you take breaks?

– How many times do we ask what
  time it is?

– What do you remember about your
  childhood?

– What do you remember when being
  a teenager?

– Have you saved an animal?

– What's not offensive?

– Are people offensive because they're hurting?

– What is said that hits home for you?

– What do you do when you wake up?

– How are you successful?

– Do you stretch in the morning?

– You know the thing you always had to have, well do you still have it, let alone use it or wear it?

– Do you warm up by the sun?

– How do you sit?

– Where does inspiration come from?

– What makes your face frown?

– How many different ways can you sit?

– Did I you just try and figure out and do the last question?

- What's dry?

- Hat or no hat?

- Have you warmed up enough?

- Why does getting warm make people sleepy?

- Does the sun or the moon have a soul?

- Do you work with what you have?

- How many holes are there?

- Where is your mindset at?

- Have you ever taken a random flight to anywhere?

- Where have you not flown to?

- What lotions do you use?

- How do you wear your hats?

- Are you demanding?

– Can you be gentle?

– How do you show your appreciation?

– What do you imagine when looking out of an airplane window?

– What are your favorite dreams?

– Do you daydream?

– What's the difference between daydreaming and imagining?

– Do you let yourself be vulnerable?

– Are you cleaner than your car?

– What corners do you cut?

– What do you lean on?

– Are you getting high?

– What is your low?

– Do you get drunk?

- Do you enjoy a glass of wine?

- Where did you move from?

- What are you not going back to?

- Who's going to save the hero?

- Could you paint something and let it go?

- Have you lost a friend?

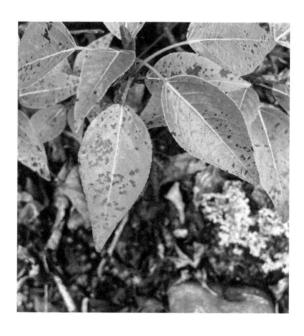

- Have you ever had to push a motorcycle or a car?

- Have you used a scale?

- Do colors contribute to mental problems?

- How many times have you taken that picture?

- How many road trips have you been on?

- Do you like to be in a relationship?

- Are you an animal person or a people person?

- Have you eaten today?

- Are you your biggest fan?

- Are you scared?

- Has your rabbit whole changed?

- What changed your rabbit whole?

- Are you good at listening?

- Have you ever been flooded with memories?

- What are you pushing through?

- Have you ever rewatched a show to only hear the music?

- What woke you up this morning?

- When's the last time you got something new?

- Do you like the sounds that are around you?

- What would you do if the internet shut down?

- Does your livelihood depend on the internet?

- What is happiness to you?

- Who are you playing for?

– What have you packed away lately?

– Can you dance?

– Where is the last place you took a walk?

– What's real to you?

– What's the point?

– Why get all this stuff or things if it's all going to break down anyway?

– Are you ever cat called?

– Who have you reached out to lately?

– Do you see anything wrong with your lifestyle?

– Are you informed?

– Do you watch the news?

– What is the most traveled road?

– When the most time traveled?

– What poisons are in your life?

– Are you observant?

– When and where is the first snowfall?

– Can you show sympathy?

– What are your excuses?

– What are your weekend plans?

– Where have you been to lately?

– Are you willing to share your dreams with a stranger?

– Have you ever stuck your head in the sand?

– How far are you willing to push things?

– Have you ever been kicked out of a place?

– If you could go back in time, would you?

– What blank pages are you starring at?

– Where do you find yourself?

– What do you want to say?

– What are you trying not to look at?

– What's inside your soul?

– How dark do you like your coffee?

– Can you see inside yourself?

– Do you remember the last restaurant you ate at?

– What symbol has the most meaning to you and why?

– Have you ever been in a car accident?

– Why does darkness mean evil?

- What's your wildest dream?

- How well do you know yourself?

- What are you nervous about?

- What are you getting tested for?

- Where's the rule book?

- What do you have to sign?

- What question do you hate?

- Have you ever tried thinking inside the box?

- Have you been in a box?

- What are your rules?

- What's the one animal you've always wanted?

- Can you stay sober from whatever it is your addictions are?

- What's the best possible things in life?

- What is the best possible scenario to live in?

- What is the best motto to live by?

- Do you know better now?

- Are you willing to bet on yourself?

- Do you want to own your own business?

- Have you ever watched a rain drop drizzle down a window?

- What does the tree of life mean to you?

- Do you wear hats?

- Have you ever written a business plan?

- What does it take to run a successful business?

- What is your success story?

- Are you stuck in a rut?

- What does it take for you to get things done?

- Are you love?

- Do you know who hates you?

- What is your focus on?

- How dedicated are you?

- Are you faithful?

- How reliable are you?

- What's in a name?

- Do you allow your name to define who you are?

- What choices have you made lately?

- What do you say when someone hiccups?

– What are you lying about?

– Have you ever called a number that was in your dream?

– Can youth teach an elder?

– Have you ever sent a love letter to yourself?

– What is your love language?

– How many books are you reading right now?

– What is it about you that made me so mad?

– What's in you, that's in me?

– What do you burden yourself with?

– What are your enjoyments?

– Have you ever stayed inside all day inside and didn't notice that you never went outside all day or night till it was over?

– What's the first things you work on in the morning, are they different every morning, do you change it up?

– Do you believe Chang is good or bad and why?

– What is it about philosophy questions that are so appealing?

– What is philosophy to you?

– Have you seen a coyote?

– Have you been followed by a coyote?

– Have you ever followed a coyote before?

– Have you gone on a spiritual walk?

– What does it mean to be spiritual to you?

– Will I ever become a successful artist let alone a businesswoman?

– What is your pain?

- Have you ever ended up with someone else's list?

- Have you ever called a random unknown number?

- What will it take for you to move forward?

- How far have you pushed some one?

- How angry have you made someone else?

- Do you type or write out your late-night thoughts?

- What would you do if you never saw a rainbow again?

- What would you do without music?

- What do you see on a daily basis?

- How do you help others?

- What do you wish you had?

- Where's your head at?

- Do you understand electricity?

- What do you want to learn more about?

- Did God make us to have his random thoughts?

- Does God have random thoughts?

- What helps you get creative?

- When's the last time God got creative?

- Did God make us so he wouldn't have to be creative anymore?

- Our we God's consciousness as a collective whole?

- What's the most stared at object/ objects?

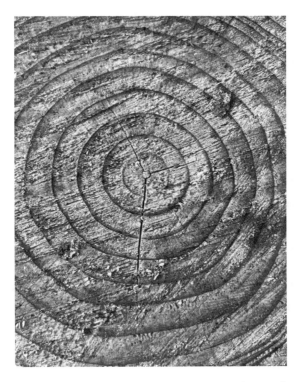

– What's the most thought of thought?

– What's the most worn shoe?

– What's the longest someone's gone
without shoes?

– Who do you think you are?

– What is your natural hair color?

– What is your eye color?

– How many surgeries have you had?

– How many names are there?

– Do you like your name?

– What's the scariest thing you've ever been through?

– How do you handle your day?

– What is it about the colors that helps people make their decisions?

– Have you ever painted?

– What hobbies do you like?

– Have you rock climbed before?

– Have you ever listened to someone else's heartbeat before?

– What's the highest you've ever flown?

- What animals have you seen?

- What animals have you touched let alone pet?

- How much do you know?

- Are you still willing to learn?

- If you already have all of the answers, then why do you ask the questions?

- Why would you want to survive the end of the world?

- What's in it for you?

- How many things have you accomplished?

- Have you ever counted how many people that you've met in a day let alone in a month?

- Are you comfortable?

- Have you gone too far?

– Are you willing to do what it takes to get you better with you?

– What are you focused on?

– What are you going through?

– Are you always where you've wanted to be?

– What have you let go of recently?

– How have you survived?

– Have you helped anyone?

– What have you been through that's unbelievable?

– Did you think you'd be best friends forever?

– What makes your world go round?

– What makes you sick?

– Do you have any stuffed animals?

– Have you ever proposed?

– Do you know how to play a musical instrument?

– How are you in a relationship?

– How do you meditate?

– Do you smudge?

– Do you like to snuggle?

– How do you feel about yoga?

– What does being sustainable mean to you?

– Have you ever had visions?

– Have you ever been on a vision quest?

– How many dreams of yours have come true?

– How many dreams are you working towards?

- What's the worst lie that you tell yourself?

- Do you trust you?

- What makes you laugh?

- What grosses you out?

- What do you miss the most?

- Do you enjoy meetings?

- What would your love story say about you?

- How well do you know the people around you? Right now, or in your past?

- Do you want to get to know them more?

- How do you remember things, what helps you?

- Have you ever let GPS help you find you?

- How do you set goals?

- How well do you finish things?

- What makes a lot of noise in your life?

- What are your problems?

- What are your excuses?

- What are your solutions?

- What are your thoughts?

- What are your options?

- What are your opinions?

- What are your ideas?

- Do you still feel like you're on the run?

- Can you be alone with your thoughts?

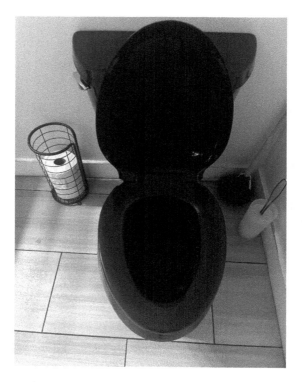

– What's one movie you've watched over a ton of times?

– Who would you stand up for?

– What are you binge watching right now?

– Could you love you more then you do right now?

– When's the last time you made a wish?

– Have you ever broken a bone?

– What's your favorite day?

– What month do you like the most?

– Who do you want back in your life?

– Do you like how you smell?

– What do you think about right before you go to bed or sleep?

– What do you think about when you wake up?

– What words do you have a hard time spelling?

– Do you like being told what to do?

– Would you like to be in charge?

– What direction are you headed in?

– Who are you watching?

– What are you caring for?

– Do you have someone watching out for you?

– What do you want to know?

– Do you know your family history?

– Have you been rewarded lately?

– What are your freedoms?

– Did you know you are beautiful?

– Do you know the history of the land in witch you live on?

– What are you born to do?

– What are you trying to do alone that you should be getting help with?

– What should you stop doing?

- What are your healthy emotions you forget to focus on the most?

- What's your growth like?

- What animals have you learned about?

- Do you know anything about rocks?

- What's plants have you learned about?

- What types of minerals do you know about?

- Are you an herbalist?

- Do you garden?

- Have you raised any animals?

- What does raising mean to you?

- Do you stand tall even when you don't want to?

- Where have you walked bare foot?

- Do you like thunderstorms?

- What's the best compliment you've ever gotten?

- What's the sweetest smell?

- Do you like lightning?

- What sound scares you?

- What sound excites you?

- What sound thrills you?

- What touch is the best feeling?

- Do you like the dark or the light?

- What side of the bed do you like to sleep on?

- What's your cozy position?

- Do you move a lot in your sleep?

- Do you move a lot in life?

- What's the thing you think you think about the most?

- What graphs have you used?

- What art have you bought?

- What do you like?

- If love is deception, then who are you fooling?

- How did you make your money?

- How did you make the day better for either yourself or someone else?

- What have you enjoyed lately?

- What goes on in your mind?

- If you could be anything, what would you be?

- If you could do anything, what would you do?

- What hurts you?

- What are you willing to do?

- What would you change?

- Why do things seem so difficult at times, then easy other times?

- Why do bees and other buzzy things think my face is a flower or me in general?

- Have you ever been open and vulnerable?

- Have you ever gone naked?

- How many plans have you made and not finished?

- When's the last time you thanked someone?

- Have you ever closed your eyes while on a walk and trusted yourself blindly?

- What diets have you tried?

– Do you always care what you look like?

– What games do you play?

– What have you not cooked?

– What are you not finishing?

– What are you dedicated to?

– What is your ideal living space?

– What do you hope to accomplish?

– Do you love the sound of birds?

– Do you like the sounds around you right now?

– What is it about you that you like?

– Can you think about what others need for a whole week, without thinking of your own?

- Have you ever stopped what you were doing immediately to help someone else?

- Have you ever helped yourself by helping someone else?

- What are your plans?

- Can you go for a swim right now, and will you?

- What's the longest you've ever looked up, can you time yourself now or maybe do it later?

- What about how long have you ever looked down?

- What's the last thing you shopped for?

- What are the most things you have owned?

- What's the most expensive thing to own?

– What's the most least expensive thing to own?

– Where do you want to live?

– Are you just settling?

– How confident are you?

– Do you like to cook or go out to eat?

– What do you like to drink the most of?

– Did you like the first book?

– Do you know who you work with?

– Do you have time for you?

– When's the last time you got away?

– Who helps you out?

– What are you trying not to do?

– What do your expressions say about you?

- What does your sense of style say about you?

- Are you the popular one?

- Who thinks you're cool, most importantly do you think your cool?

- Do you have friends to reach out to?

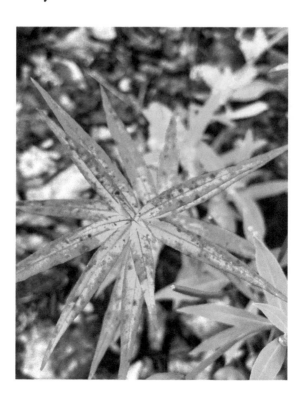

– When's the last time you changed something in your life?

– Have you changed a light bulb lately?

– Is the spotlight on you?

– Can you handle the spotlight?

– Do you judge people by what they are wearing?

– When's the last time you read a newspaper or have you ever read the newspaper?

– Would you read the newspaper for a week or a month, could you, do it?

– What are your commitments?

– Do you leave your house to escape your world or go to your house to escape the world or a bit of both?

– Can you see who you truly are?

– Who is that?

– What's the hardest job you've ever had?

– Did you ever think you would ever do what you've done so far in life?

– Can you go on a date with a stranger?

– What will help you get further in life?

– Are you a leader or a follower?

– What do you not mention let alone bring up in conversations?

– Who pushes you to do better in life?

– Are you struggling?

– Do you know you will be okay?

– Is life just a bunch of phases like how the moon goes through them?

– What is your ideal life?

– Do you want something different?

– Are you willing to be better?

– What can you do?

– What have you studied?

– What colors are you attracted to?

– What do you know about the world?

– What is it about seeking in life that is helpful?

– Where do you find the most solace in life?

– What's the last song you listened to?

– What was the last flower you smelled?

– Have you ever stopped in the middle of a crowd and looked up, and if not, would you?

– What makes you spin?

- Do you like the sound of buzzy things?

- What attracts you to the people you know?

- Do you like meetings?

- Do you like work?

- Would you show your answers to someone else?

- What is your connection like?

- Have you ever been homeless?

- When did you get your first car?

- Do you remember your first pair of shoes?

- Do you remember the first thing you bought all on your own?

- Where are you taking you?

- What does beauty mean to you?

– What do you see when you look at me?

– Once one dies can one still feel cold and hot?

– Do you see things differently now that you have changed?

– Do you know where you are going?

– Do you want to continue to change for the better?

– What's different?

– How do you look at grass?

– When's the last time you took a walk in the forest?

– What's stoping you?

– Do you like taking photos?

– Who do you love?

– What's subtle in your life?

- Where do you begin your day?

- Have you ever talked with the dead?

- Who have you offended?

- What's the last flight you took and where was it to?

- Are you trustworthy?

- Would you show your enemies love and kindness?

- Do you know who truly supports you?

- How rich are you?

- How many ways are there to figure things out?

- What are your true colors?

- How do you see things?

- What is it about thinking that's got you thinking more or thinking less?

– How much stuff do you bring with you?

– When was your last check up?

– Do you appreciate people in your life?

– What boarders have you put up?

– Have you evolved?

– Has your creativity surpassed what you thought you could ever do?

– Do you tell people your weight?

– How do people react to you?

– What is your reaction to their reaction?

– Are you a nice person all the time?

– Are you startled easily?

– What are your traumas?

– What are your breakthroughs?

– At what points in life have you reached the top?

– Did you appreciate the process or the journey?

– We're you happy when you finally finished what it was you were working on?

– How much more do you have to get done?

– Are you on edge?

– Is the sun out today?

– Can you wiggle your toes or blink your eyes or maybe take a deep breath?

– Can you cross one eye and roll the other one?

– Did you try it, was it weird?

– Why do things go blurry when we cross our eyes?

– Do you even understand from which level of launguage you even speak?

– What does understand mean if the launguage is lost?

– Do you see white dots every now and then?

– What is it about love language that gets people lost?

– What are you confused about?

– How do you find your way back?

– What have you lost recently?

– What are you receiving in your life right now?

– How does connection start?

– How is connection lost?

- What are the bright colors in your life?

- What's the tallest building you've seen in real life?

- Why is white considered angelic?

- Who decided what the colors were and why?

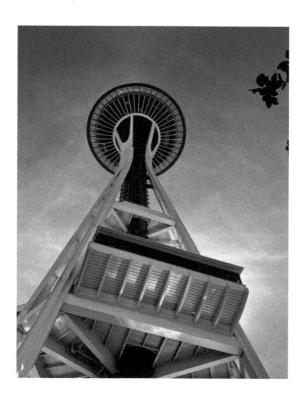

– Have you made a blanket?

– Are you disorganized?

– What defines organized?

– Can you be cluttered and still be organized?

– How many opinions do you have, have you ever written them all down?

– If you could swim in the sky, would you?

– Where have you gone swimming?

– What's the coldest water you've ever touched?

– What's the hottest water you've ever touched?

– Have you ever had hot wax poured on you?

– What was your childhood dream?

– What are your dreams now?

– What was good about growing up?

– Do you see the light where the darkness used to be?

– Have you realized that to feed both wolves is better than just one?

– What animal did you want to be growing up?

– Can you skip rocks?

– Do you like looking at your reflection?

– What are you enjoying right now?

– What have you been giving away lately?

– What's on your shelves?

– What are you having a hard time getting rid of?

- Can you handle bugs crawling on you?

- Do you reject you?

- How many smelly things do you have?

- Do you like every sound you hear?

- What is your ideal temperature?

- Why did you move to where you are?

- Are you iconic?

- What are you trying to make it in?

- What's your ideal day?

- What are you teaching others?

- What do you find morbid?

- What are you remorseful for?

- What are you looking for?

– Do you like the wind?

– Did you turn off the lights in the house when you left?

– How are you saving time?

– What are guardians to you?

– Who is brave to you?

– Do you make the love of your life carry all of the things or do you carry some with them?

– Do you trust someone based off of the way they are dressed?

– What's a constant in your life?

– How do you like your hair?

– Who are you having a hard time letting go of?

– Why do we always think it's about us?

- When's the last time you went on a date?

- How many people do you meet up with in a day let alone in a week?

- Do you tend to agree with everything and everyone to avoid conflict?

- What kind of art do you see in nature?

- What's your favorite drink/drinks?

- What outfit do you wear the most?

- What health problems do you have?

- Have you ever climbed to the top of a tree?

- Have you climbed a mountain?

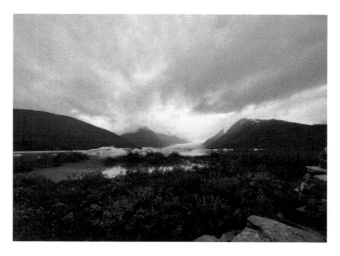

– If getting things done helps feel
accomplished, then why does it feel
like nothing is ever finished and the
list only gets longer?

– What's bittersweet to you but sweet
to someone else?

– Could you go around and ask other
people these questions?

– Is anything ever a for sure thing?

– Why do we continue to reach out to
people that don't reach out to us?

- What's the most sought-after plant in the world?

- What tree produces the most oxygen?

- What have you not experienced yet?

- What are you doing that your doctors don't want you to do?

- What are you shy about?

- Do you care for any plants?

- What does staying away mean to you?

- Do dreams stem from nightmares?

- Who doesn't love a good break up movie?

- Who are you done talking to?

- What's one thing you wish you didn't have to do anymore?

- Do you like yelling at people? If not, why do you keep doing it?

- Why do you keep on with your rude demeanor?

- Do you appreciate what people do for you and do you let them know?

- Do you always add things for people to do or do you actually enjoy their company once in a while?

- What is it about having to do stuff that gets on people's nerves?

- What if clouds were edible?

- What are your reservations?

- What are your risks?

- Would you bike somewhere to ask a stranger a question and not just any questions but possibly a life altering one?

- Where have you biked to?

– Who do you hope shows up?

– What do you want to be working on?

– What sounds weird to you?

– Who would be the last person you would want to talk to?

– Why do you take so long to respond?

– What is it about the human race that has to have companionship?

– Why don't coffee shops have books?

– What's going on with the creative mind?

– Where are you going today?

– What journey have you not taken yet and why not?

– Who's always there for you?

– What is it about waiting that annoys most people?

– Have you ever tried a dating app and if so, what was your experience?

– Do you like the sun or shade better?

– What flowers are edible?

– What flowers are poisonous?

– Have you ever been poised by accident, either by yourself or someone else?

– What are you finding out?

– Why do you even keep going backwards?

– What bugs you the most?

– What's in a splatter?

– What does it take for you to get ready for the day?

– How many people could you share a hotel room with?

- How much pain does a tree go through as it grows?

- What are the consequences of your actions from today?

- What ripple effects happened due to what you have done?

- Do you remember the first question?

- Do you remember the first answer?

- Do you remember what baffles you the most and why?

- What's the one thing that you believe has altered your life completely and why?

- What's the one thing that would make your life better?

- Do you like how you feel right now and why?

- Are you happy that certain things are gone from your life? What are they and why?

- Do you like bugs?

- Do you smile at random people?

- How many people do you give compliments to in a day, let alone in a week?

- Are your kind to your neighborhood/ neighbors?

- What are your reasons for doing what you're doing right now?

- What pain are you in at the moment?

- What is the most pleasant you've ever felt?

- What cars have you not driven or driven in?

- What flowers have you yet to see in real life?

– Would you work on something to save your life or someone else's life?

– What music calms you down?

– What are you not ready to let go of yet?

– What's cluttering in your life right now?

– What's the clutter in your head?

– Do you believe in what you're doing?

– Do you spark hope in other's lives and how?

– What makes things clear?

– How do you make or create things in your life?

– Do you always want more?

– Could you go without, what you have, why or why not?

- How could you simplify your life?

- What would you downsize in your life and in the world?

- Do you seek nature?

- Do you believe nature seeks us?

- How healthy do you eat and drink?

- Have you ever been busted by a random friend for being on a dating app?

- Do people ask you for guidance?

- Do you have a hard time sleeping at night, why?

- What's your ideal life like?

- What's your most ideal piece of art?

- Are you usually warmer or colder in temperature?

- How much water do you drink in a day?

- How much caffeine do you have in a day?

- What games do you play?

- Are you invested in yourself?

- Would you seek treatment if you needed it?

- What is it about treatment that scares people?

- Why do people want a solution then balk on the work to get it?

- What message do you carry around with you?

- What message do you spread to help others out?

- How long can you sit in a room by yourself for?

- Are you at peace with yourself?

- Who came up with plastic plants?

- Do you prefer plastic, paper, glass, cardboard or cloth when packing your groceries?

- Can a home really be happy or are the people happier when out of it?

- What would you never do?

- What do you really want to stop doing?

- Who do you walk with?

- What's your favorite exercise?

- What's your favorite experience?

- What's your favorite product?

- Do you wear glasses?

- What kinds of shoes do you have?

- What is your favorite pair of shoes to wear and why?

- Do you have a favorite outfit and why?

- Do the change of seasons bother you or do you love them why or why not?

- Have you ever done your own hair, how did it turn out and did you like or love it?

- What do you clean in your life, and do you find enjoyment out of it?

- Have you ever planted a tree?

- Have you ever seen things grow up around you?

- How focused are you?

- How determined are you?

- How much detail do you pay attention to?

– Have you noticed the changes around you?

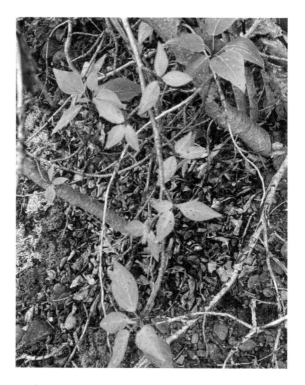

– What's repetitive in your life?

– What have you dreamed about lately?

– Where are you starting at today?

- Can you take things away from God?

- What have you witnessed?

- Can you swim?

- Have you ever swam in your clothing?

- Have you ever drowned?

- What have been your close calls?

- Have you ever raced anyone?

- What does workforce mean to you?

- Are you yourself in your backyard?

- Do you hide away at your own home?

- Do you like peace and quiet in the mornings?

- How do you like to watch movies?

- Would you ever write a book?

- What do you find funny that others say or do?

- Do you really care what's going on around you and why or why not?

- How many trees are planted each year?

- Have you ever looked into a plant you found on a hike?

- What's a color you can't look at?

- Have you ever walked on the beach and picked up shells?

- Are you doing things for you or someone else?

- Where's your head at today?

- What's the worst physiological mind trick to do to yourself?

- Do you enjoy hammocks?

– What was the best day you have ever had?

– Who's the bright spot in your life?

– Do you trust people?

– Do you know what gets rid of bugs?

– Why all the secrecy?

– Do you inspire growth?

– Do you get ready for you or other people?

– How do you get ready and how long does it take?

– Are you okay with who you're around?

– Do you get others to feel comfortable or uncomfortable?

– Do you mean it when you ask how someone is feeling?

- Where do you like to go swimming?

- What's your grand adventure?

- Do you like hide and seek?

- What is it about surprises that some people like and others don't?

- What's the last compliment you got?

- What's your favorite past time?

- Do you do what your asked?

- Are you available?

- Are you ready for what's to come next, whatever that might be?

- Are you okay with the unknown?

- What is it about electronics that bugs some and gets others happy?

- Why don't electronics work for me right all the time?

– What's going on in the world right now?

– How do you escape?

– What is it about puzzling situations that are so fascinating?

– Would you be okay if all the art in the world disappeared?

– What if your favorite thing disappeared, what would you do?

– What are you driven to do?

– What have you become?

– What are you backing away from?

– What are you done with doing all the time?

– Are you ready to change your eating habits?

– What is it that makes you want to change?

– How do you function when society isn't?

– How do you feel about writing your thoughts down?

– What makes you sleepy?

– How long can you sit for?

– How long can you stand?

– What's the heaviest thing you can carry and for how long can you carry it for?

– What languages can you understand?

– What did you notice on this trip that you didn't notice last time?

– What colors do you see when your eyes are closed?

– What do you volunteer for?

– Do you enjoy what you eat?

– Have you ever missed your flight?

– Do you know why mistakes happen?

– Why did you sleep in today and not yesterday?

– What are your next travel plans?

– Do you like to travel alone?

– How do you pack your things?

– How many trains have your ridden on?

– How many train tracks go unused?

– How many earthquakes are there in a year?

– Have you ever had to have surgery on your birthday?

– How do you like to travel?

– What is it about traveling that you like the most?

- Do you like goodbyes or hellos more?

- Have you ever touched a glacier?

- Are there any mistakes in my last book?

- Do you like the person that your becoming?

- Could you defend yourself if you had to?

- What kind of jewelry do you wear?

- Are you loud or quiet?

- Where did you come from?

- How much baggage are you carrying around with you?

- What do you need to unload, yet won't?

- Would you plaster your face for all to, see?

- How would you rate yourself, as a child, as a teenager, as adult, and right now?

- How do you perceive beauty?

- What would you like to happen?

- What's the most pain you've ever been in?

- How long has your flight been delayed before?

- What emergencies have you been through?

- What is delightful to you?

- What is delicious to you?

- Have you changed any habits lately?

- Are you willing to make a difference and also put forth the action to make a change?

- Are we moving?

– What was that?

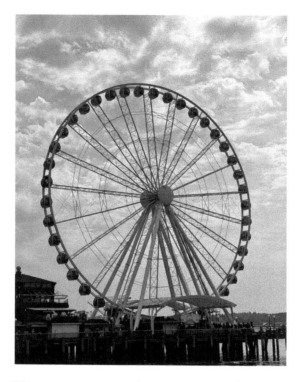

– How many mushrooms are there?

– How many berries are there?

– How much water is in a rain drop?

– Does weather disrupt your day?

- Are you in a hurry?

- How many numbers are there?

- Could you survive without your phone?

- Could you survive without electricity?

- Have you paddle boarded?

- Have you surfed?

- Have you swam with the dolphins or the turtles?

- Are you ready for the day ahead of you?

- Have you seen any standup comedians?

- What does being polite look like to you?

- Is your Brain playing tricks on you?

– Would you just pick up everything
and move to somewhere random,
where you knew no one and start
completely over/new?

– Are you going to stop doing that
habit yet?

– Why haven't you gone on your
dream vacation yet?

– Are we moving yet?

– Can you curl your tongue, crinkle
your nose and cross your eyes all at
the same time?

– Where would you rather be?

– What's your favorite candy?

– How much water do you drink?

– How much food do you eat?

– What's the rainiest place?

– What's the driest place?

- What's the longest book ever written?

- What's the shortest book ever written?

- How well do you know the people around you?

- What do you like to show people?

- What do you like to talk to people about?

- What noises can you make?

- Do you twiddle your thumbs?

- Do you respect other's boundaries?

- Do you respect your own boundaries?

- How nice are you to you?

- Food or water?

- Air or fire?

- Earth or space?

- Crowds or forest?

- What's your preferred way of paying for things?

- What's your ideal person to be around?

- What's it like being you?

- Describe what you're looking at right now in five words, lol just kidding make it as long or short as you like, well what do you see?

- What did you decide to wear today and why?

- How much have things changed since you were a child?

- Why is it that we lose sight of our childhood dreams as we get older?

- How many questions were in my last book?

- How many are in this one?

- Are there any mistakes in this one?

- Do you like airplane food or hospital food?

- What diets have you tried?

- What diet are you doing now?

- Would you all of a sudden change career given the opportunity?

- What would you do if everything was paid for?

- How do you handle someone when they are freaking out?

- Are you judgmental?

- What are you snacking on?

- How silly can you get?

- Do you know that smiles are just as contagious as yawns or are they?

- What are some fun facts that you know?

- What are some weird random facts that you know?

- Do you know anything about the state in which you live in?

- What does Lady Liberty represent to you?

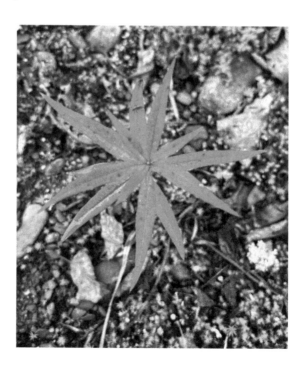

- How does other actions affect your behavior?

- Have you ever been hunting?

- Have you bought furs or hides before?

- What's your perspective on hunting?

- How do you feel about people who wear furs or use them for blankets let alone shoes?

- How many animals are there?

- Have all animals been discovered?

- Have you ever stayed in a cabin and if so for how long?

- Do you like ice?

- Have you done meditation lately?

- What color is the sky now?

- Are you seeing right?

- What have you spilt lately?

- Have you had company over in a while?

- If you could visit anyone you wanted, who would it be and why?

- Did you wake up on the right side of life?

- Did you wake up on the right side of the bed?

- Do you love yourself enough to go to work also show that love to your coworkers and to those around you?

- How do you carry yourself?

- How well do handle yourself under pressure?

- Do you realize you helped me with more questions?

- Do you like to eat breakfast?

– Do you like to stay in a hotel?

– Are you working right now and do people not realize that's what you're doing?

– Can you go to work in cozy clothes?

– Who have you said good morning to lately and did you know them?

– Do you like your options for what you have to eat?

– Have you gotten lost lately?

– Do you like the patterns that you see around you?

– How many shapes are in a room?

– What have you done for fun for you lately?

– Boxes or bags?

– What is your ideal living place?

– Do you like houses or apartments?

– Can you hear, ok?

– Can you see things that are in front of you?

– How well can you walk?

– Why is the process of writing a book longer than reading one?

– Do you let other's go ahead of you?

– What's the rudest you've ever been?

– What's the kindest you've ever been?

– How well do you work with others?

– Do you pluck your eyebrows?

– How do you brush your teeth?

– Where are you from?

– Do you have an accent, and does it make you sound mean or nice?

- Do you have whiskers that you gotta pluck?

- Do you have roadside assistance?

- Do you have a way to help yourself?

- What does your spirit say?

- How do you draw?

- Do you hear the calling?

- What does Mother Earth tell you?

- How do you speak to the universe?

- How well do you treat Mother Earth?

- Are you so encompassed in yourself that you forget to wish others well?

- Have you ever showed up to early somewhere by accident?

- Have you ever showed up way to early on purpose?

- How tired do you feel?

- Was the date worth it?

- What's the best date you've been on?

- Who are you waiting on?

- Can you get into deep thought even if you are foggy brained?

- What should you have brought with you?

- What is it that you're always forgetting to bring?

- What are you waiting to purchase?

- Do you have people that hope you travel safely?

- Who cares about you?

- Do people tear others down due to them being jealous, do they realize even being nice is still tearing down?

- Have you ever made travel goals?

- What's bugging you right now?

- Why do things have to change?

- What's the longest you've stayed at an airport?

- What things have you been getting rid of lately?

- Are you willing to wait?

- Do you scare people?

- Do you help people smile?

- Are you helpful when needed?

- How quite can you be?

- Are you careful with the words you speak?

- Do you allow what others say to affect you in any way?

- How many fairs have you been to?

- How many rides have you ridden?

- Are you in the right spot?

- How much do you charge for your time?

- How do your feet feel?

- Do you have what it takes to get you through what you're going through?

- What are you excited for?

- Who's the last stranger you talked with, and did you become friends?

- How many key chains do you have?

- Are you willing to let go of everything?

- Are you happy for you?

- What did you celebrate last for?

- What are you promoting?

- What's one thing you know about your neighbor they don't know you know?

- What's one thing you would like your neighbor to quit doing?

- Are you friendly with your neighbor?

- How many cups of coffee have you had in one day?

- Do you do yard sales?

- Can you sleep in the cold?

- Have you been stood up lately and do you let it affect you?

- Who is the who of all who's in the know today?

- Are any of these questions baffling yet?

– What's been the one that's got you thinking the longest so far, between this book and the first book?

– Will some of our answers be the same, I wonder how many?

– Will we finish around the same time?

– Did you realize there were so many questions?

– Are you one that has to have all the answers?

– Do you like puzzles?

– Do you like riddles?

– What continues and never really ends?

– Where do shapes come from?

– Who came up with shapes?

– Why is one shape more appealing than the other's?

– Does the ether have a master?

– Is coffee your master?

– Do you have wings?

– Have you gotten new tattoos since the last one?

– Do you walk bare foot when camping?

– How do you like to camp?

– Where do you like to go camping?

– Do you walk bare foot in the city?

– What time do you have your first cup of coffee?

– How do you function in society?

– Do you have someone that you tell everything to?

– What's it like to be alone for one's whole life?

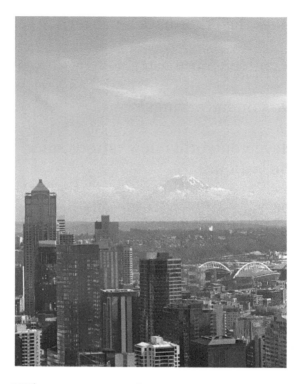

- What conversations are going on around you?

- Do you like the temperature right now?

- What's crazy to you?

- How long have you been waiting for?

- How long do you think it takes to write a book?

- What events have you been attending lately?

- Who are you supporting today?

- Do you ever just wash your hair in the sink?

- Who do you live with, and do you get along, why or why not?

- What needs to change?

- How many different types of hats are there?

- How many different ways are there to keep things cold?

- How many different things are there to keep things hot?

- What keeps you going?

- How many different types of chairs are there?

- How do you sit?

- How do you meditate?

- How do you pray or do you?

- Do you exercise?

- Do you except how the world is right now?

- Are you demanding?

- What was the last picture you took?

- What have you been working on lately?

- Am I running out of questions?

- Will I be able to have all the answers lol?

- Do you worry and stress over things you have no control over?

– Can you let things go?

– Are you determined when you set a goal?

– Do you cross your legs, are you doing it right now and did you know that it's a bad habit?

– What's the last time you had a really good laugh?

– Is anyone staring at you or are they all just looking at their devices, did you just look around?

– Is there a breeze blowing where you're at?

– Are there any clouds?

– What color are the trees, or should I say leaves right now?

– Have you ever really looked at the bark of a tree before or the lines on a leaf?

- What details in life have you paid attention to and what was it that intrigued you to do that at the time?

- Are you running late?

- Have you ever gone rock collecting?

- Have you ever been bird watching?

- Have you been on a scavenger hunt?

- What do you hold dear to you?

- Would you write out your life story and would you publish it?

- What is it about groups of people that bothers you?

- What have you admitted lately?

- Are you willing to make things right?

- What kind of contact do you have with others?

- Can you make it back?

– Are you finally seeing the things you
never saw before?

– Are you talking more about the dead
or the living or of the ones you know
either way?

– Does religion bother you?

– What's the longest you've kept your
phone turned off?

– What is medicine to you?

– What is your medicine?

– What are your wounds?

– How do you heal?

– What is it about being free that
people are afraid of?

– What are your feather colors?

– What's flying for you?

– Is your drum beat steady?

– What are you listening to right now?

– What are you wasting?

– Are you sensible?

– What's being on the verge mean to you?

– What are you finding?

– What would you rather be doing?

– Have you found your purpose yet?

– What is real talk or communication to you?

– Are you involved within a community?

– What does community represent to you?

– Does the tongue and mind really connect or are there times they are disconnected?

- Do you have a good memory?

- How many memories do you have stored away in your brain?

- How do you find your inspiration?

- What is it if not for the whole?

- What are the things to come?

- Do you use visual aids?

- Do you need examples for an explanation over anything?

- What is tangible to you?

- What's at stake for you?

- Are you having a hard time focusing or concentrating?

- Who are better men or women?

- What's a better paycheck to you?

- Are you living fearfully?

– How long have you gone without TV?

– What are you caught up in?

– Are you into the new trend?

– What are your fantasies?

– What is your ego doing, is it in the way of accomplishing your dreams?

– What melodies are playing in your head?

– Do you pay attention to the other times?

– Do you gather with others?

– Are you nervous?

– Are you wasting your hate?

– What emotions do you waste?

– Do you get creative?

- Are you as amused as you used to be at the things you used to go to?

- Are you amused at what you did today, why or why not?

- Did you know that squirrels eat more than just nuts?

- Have you ever just sat and enjoyed a meal with a squirrel before?

- Do you like the smell of a new magazine?

- Do you take responsibility for your own actions?

- Are you done looking at others faults and ready to fix your own as well as ready to move forward?

- Who hasn't made a mistake?

- What's the cleanest place in the world?

- Have you been horseback riding?

- Why am I now ready to be adventurous again?

- What's the longest you've had a pair of pants or a piece of clothing?

- What does by the seaside mean to you?

- What animal represents the most meaning to you?

- Did you sleep like a baby last night?

- How long can you wait till you have coffee?

- Do you make a mess when making your coffee?

- How clean is your coffee maker?

- How quickly do you respond to people?

- How soft is your toilet seat?

- Do you like cushions?

– Have you ever thought of going to
  the store to read the Hallmark cards
  to make your day better, let alone
  have tried it and have you bought
  one to send to someone to hopefully
  make their day better?

– Do you realize the artist that you
  just commented on their artwork is
  sitting right next to you?

– Can you paint what I paint?

– Can you sell the things you create?

– How many helicopter pilots get sick
  and tired of flying?

– Do birds get fed up with flight and
  want to not fly anymore?

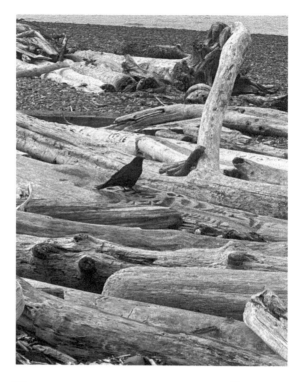

– Do you ever not want to walk
anymore?

– Are you overwhelmed with what you
have accomplished?

– Will I ever go work for someone
else?

– Have you ever sat on a thumb tack?

- What are you working harder at?

- What box are you trying to fit in?

- What system works best for you?

- What are you ready to work for?

- What is fortitude to you and what are you willing to do to attempt to attain it?

- What is your pain today or what is hurting you?

- Are you going around being mad about things in your past, are you ready to let them go?

- Have you ever been to a book signing/event?

- What do you pray for?

- Are your affairs in order?

- What principles do you live by?

- What do you think the universe is taking care of for you?

- What is it that you express in your life?

- What's happening in your life right now that's unexpected?

- What is your why?

- Can you do things on your own or do you have to meet up with others?

- Can you see the shadows of the sun's rays?

- Can you see the diversity of the yellows in a field?

- Do you do things to gain attention for yourself or to help others feel better about themselves or a bit of both?

- Did you just see something you didn't want to?

– What is natural beauty mean to you?

– Can you slow down and take it easy?

– What are you in a rush for or are you in a rush?

– What did you use to do as a child that you loved?

– Have you ever cut up a fresh pineapple before?

– Do you drive scared?

– Do you drive and if so, what do you drive, is it what you've always wanted to drive?

– How many of your childhood dreams have come true, are you still working on making them come true why or why not?

– What do you pray for?

– What can you not go through ever again?

- What is your adventurous life?

- Who are you being kind to toady?

- What have you been suggesting to others lately?

- What people in your life scare you the most?

- What people in your life do you love the most?

- What does be social mean to you?

- How do you go and meet people?

- What is fulfilling to you?

- What are you repairing today?

- What does be solid mean to you?

- Are you solid?

- Are you grateful in your life?

- What are you contributing to?

- What do you write about?

- Do you keep your mouth shut or do you speak your mind?

- Have you been to a comedy club?

- What's taking you forever to accomplish?

- What do you think is going downhill?

- What were some of your firsts?

- Are you afraid to pray?

- What is your head spinning about today?

- What do you think is easy that may be harder for others?

- Have you ever sung with the birds?

- Are you being reckless?

- Do you think about God?

– What does God mean to you?

– What do you share with others?

– Are you a secret away from hiding away from yourself?

– What are your truths that you lie to yourself about?

– How many insecurities do you have?

– Did you know that just because your mind tricks you that you can turn around and trick It?

– How do you work best?

– What are you currently working on that you think will better your life and possibly help others?

– Do you hope to become better each day or at least better than you were in the past?

– Will this book ever see the light of day?

- Will I finish the third book and how long will it take me to write it?

- Do you know what your neighbors do for a living?

- Would you invite your neighbors over for dinner or tea?

- What is it about certain people that annoys you?

- Is the air quality better where you are?

- What is your skin care regimen?

- Do you soak in the sun?

- Do you do yoga?

- What religions have you looked into let alone been a part of?

- What does spirit realm mean to you?

- What does give up hope mean to you?

- Do you clip your own nails, or do you get them done by a professional?

- Have you ever taken care of a pine tree?

- What's your newfound love?

- What do you best connect with?

- Do you use a compass and what do you use it for, and what is the last direction you were headed in that you used it for?

- What's the freshest fruit you've ever tasted?

- Have you ever had home grown food?

- Did you know that questions never change, they can be reworded, it's the answers that change over time?

- Do you want someone else's job?

- What do you want from yourself?

– Do you know what you dream of?

– Have you ever stared into a spider's web?

– What's the last spiritual journey that you took and what was it like?

– Are you intimate?

– Have you ever felt back pain?

– Do you like the sound of kitties purring?

– I think kitties go crazy, so we don't have to, do you?

– Have you ever taken a muscle relaxer?

– What's been the best day so far?

– How well do you handle physical pain?

– Are you okay around other people when you're in pain?

- Why no food or drinks before surgeries?

- What's your favorite holiday?

- Do lights bother you?

- What is it about little square lights that intrigues people?

- Do you have a heated vest?

- How well do you handle doing a bunch of things all at once?

- Do you like your laugh?

- Do you like your situation right now?

- What are you not letting others know?

- What do you text the most?

- Who do you call the most?

- Do you believe the universe saves you from certain situations?

- Do you pay attention to your spirit animals?

- What does your spirit animals say to you?

- Do you listen to what your body is telling you?

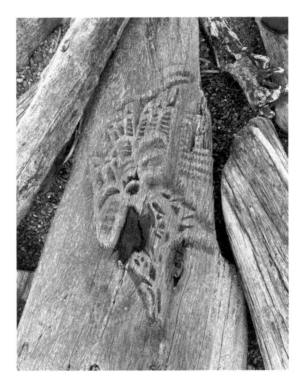

- What are you capable of?

- Do you congratulate yourself
  on the big things and the small
  accomplishments?

- Are you willing to release yourself
  from your own shackles?

- Black bird, black bird what is it that
  you see?

- Do you fight for you?

- Would you sacrifice your beauty to
  save the life of another?

- Have you ever researched your own
  medical information?

- Have you ever put together all your
  medical files?

- What do you keep losing focus on?

- What is distracting you from your
  goals?

- Are you hungry?

– Have you had coffee yet?

– Are you good at math?

– Are you good at writing?

– What instructions have you missed?

– Do you feel confident in your job?

– Why am I trying to get rid of some
   pain and not others if it's so pleasing?

– What products are you wasting?

– How much products get wasted?

– What do you wash?

– Do you have a dream catcher?

– What are you studying?

– Is your reality sweet to you?

– What's bittersweet to you, not the
   definition just life?

– What are you moving away from?

– What cultures are you learning from?

– Are you rejoicing anything right now?

– Are you connecting to what you really want to be connected to?

– Yes, or no?

– What signs are you paying attention to?

– Plurality, what does this mean to you and how does it affect you in your life?

– What are you eating and is it helping in your life and those around you?

– Are you rising up to the occasion?

– Will this book ever be published?

– Will my first book sell a bunch?

– Will my first book help out others?

– What are your hopes and dreams just for today?

– Does your clock need a new battery?

– Do you add to people's happiness?

– Do you hold others hostage with what you share?

– What's it like letting go of one and holding on to the other?

– Do you know how to help those with desperation?

– How does one harvest tree sap?

– How many different kinds of tree saps are there or are there different kinds?

– What's your chi like?

– Do you have a favorite hoodie?

- Is there a question that is not question marked?

- When's the last time you enjoyed the morning sun?

- Would you wear random cloths out in public that you normally wouldn't wear?

- What do you keep around that helps you to remember things?

- What are you scratching?

- How many published authors go to their local libraries?

- Whose permission are you seeking?

- What are you milking in your life?

- Have you seen someone choke before?

- Are you growing anything?

- Do you have animals to take care of?

– What was your favorite flower growing up and is it the same as now?

– Are you getting done what you wanted to?

– When's the last time you went to a sweat lodge?

– When was your last spirit walk?

– Do you like to sleep in the morning?

– What states have you been to?

– How do you take your coffee?

– How many filters are there?

– How much coffee do you drink?

– Do you call people back or do you forget to?

– Are you grateful?

– Are you graceful?

– Are you graced?

– Are you okay with your past?

– Do you use your past to help others?

– Do you like the sound of birds?

– Do you wear shorts in the fall?

– How do you stay warm?

– Do you warm up your car?

– What state of mind does it take to
reach ultimate peace?

– Have you ever been in utter silence?

– Are you startled easily?

– Are you ok?

– What did you see last?

– Have you been blocked before?

– Who have you let go out of your life?

- Are you accepting?

- Are you accomplished?

- Are you actually doing anything for you today?

- What is it that you can get in your life now that you are not looking at all these things you don't have or want?

- Are the things you want in life the things you need and what are they?

- What's the best way for you to get a new job?

- What are your habits?

- Do you show up early or late?

- How do you get a cat to clean their butt?

- How many times are you willing to go through something?

– Have you ever been in a parade?

– Have you been to a parade?

– What have you fixed?

– Do you drink juice and if so what's your favorite juice?

– Have you ever burnt a turkey?

– What have you burnt in the oven?

– What things took you a while to learn how to cook correctly or at least to cook the way you love them?

– Do you know what you want?

– How many meetings do you go to?

– How many different kinds of meetings are there?

– Do you feel important?

– Do kitties like to purr?

- Are their different types of purrs or are they all the same?

- Are you ready to see the truth and to do the work to seek it?

- Did you realize that you are doing that right now?

- Do you have your phone on silent most of the time?

- How many alarms do you have to get you up in the morning?

- Where are your chill spots?

- Do you still write letters to people?

- What do you hope to help someone with today?

- Have you been inspired lately?

- When's the last time you slept over at someone else's house?

- When's the last time someone cooked for you?

- When's the last time you cooked for someone else?

- Do you realize that there are a lot of people with similar looks?

- Who do you get critical over?

- What do you criticize?

- What is crucial to you and why?

- Where do you store you stuff in your house and is it organized?

- Do you drive irrationally?

- What gets you to take a deep breath to chill?

- What raises your eyebrows?

- Have you ever people watched those in front of a liquor store?

- Did you finally notice what was different where you are and how things are alternated between summer and fall?

- Still a long way to go isn't there?

- Do you like what you see in the reflection?

- If you had a name brand, what would you call it?

- What's one thing on your phone that is so funny that you have to do?

- Have you ever said a predictive text to someone?

- Have you ever done a whole predictive text and then sent it to someone as a joke?

- Have you ever seen the sun or moon in an eclipse?

- What would you call your style?

– What does comfort zone mean to you?

– What is comfortable to you?

– What is the most meaningful thing someones done for you?

– Are you still going out there for yourself to get better and to help others or are you starting to isolate?

– What is it about to many people that gets my anxiety going?

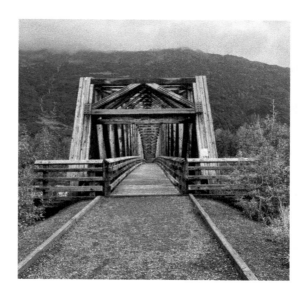

– When is the last time you filled out an application?

– Do you walk barefoot?

– Have you ever stepped on a wasp barefoot?

– How long do wasps live?

– Are you ready for the season?

– What are you not okay with?

– What have you been doing that's not okay?

– Whose approval are you after?

– What's courageous to you?

– Do you give your opinion even when you're not asked?

– Do you still act like a child?

– Have you grown up yet?

- What's does it means to be childlike and to adult at the same time?

- Have you ever spaced off into the tree branches?

- Do animals wild and non-wild get close to you?

- How connected are you?

- How good are you at hiding?

- Are you more of a relaxer or a get things done kind of person?

- What was abnormal to you about your childhood?

- What were your likes and dislikes about your childhood?

- What have you enjoyed about your life growing up?

- Did you at some point have to turn your life around due to some choices you made, what happened?

- What's your life story?

- Do you ever want to forgive yourself?

- Will you forgive those around you?

- Are you hopeful for the present moment?

- Have you ever seen a nest of mosquitoes disturbed?

- What are you doing after this?

- Who is your idol?

- What are you attracted to?

- How much noise can you handle?

- Do you like to decorate?

- Do you like how your place looks?

- Do you want to have a changed behavior about things around you?

- Are you willing to see things differently?

- What's the most tattoos someone has gotten in one session?

- What's the most pain that the human body can go through?

- Have you ever slept in a place with wild tigers or any other wild animals that were loose?

- What does natural order mean to you?

- Do you say a lot of things that you're going to do and really, you're just saying them, with no intention of doing them?

- What are your intentions when getting into a relationship, dating or otherwise?

- How quickly does your calendar fill up?

- What season colors do you like the most?

- What do you carry around with you physically and mentally?

- Would you open up your own office, if you haven't already, what and where would it be?

- How personal do you get?

- Are you grateful?

- What words do you use that others don't use?

- How often are you available for yourself?

- How often are you honestly available for others?

- How important is your time?

- What is it about procrastinating that is so appealing?

– Would you call you to talk if given the chance?

– What opportunities have you been missing out on due to your own fears?

– Do loud noises startle you?

– Do you give out compliments?

– Have you ever played baseball and if not will you, given the chance?

– Do you have bad breath?

– Does traffic bother you?

– Are your lips chapped?

– Is your skin dry?

– Do you wear sunglasses?

– What's your favorite thing to wear?

– What do you stash away?

- Would you give away your answers
  for the world to see?

- Is there controversy in your life?

- How do you distinguish between
  a turtle and elephant by which one
  goes the slowest or how long which
  one has lived the longest?

- Is all life falling apart or is it slowly
  being put back together?

- Gold or silver?

- Backwards or forwards?

- Past or present?

- Truth or lies.

- Pain or cover up?

- What are the things that are
  inevitable in life?

- What does life mean to you?

– Do you take suggestions as if you have no other choice?

– Would you give away all your money?

– Would you give all your stuff away?

– How does one start over?

– Do you care if you're on speakerphone?

– Do you have any privacy?

– What is your peace like?

– Do you have any boundaries, and do you stick to them?

– What's permanent in life?

– How many structures are there?

– How many statues are there?

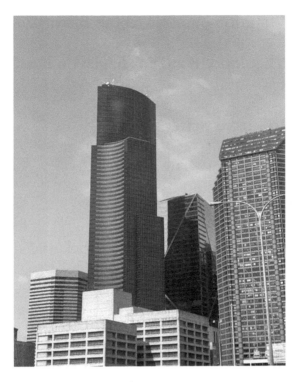

– Have you ever burnt sage?

– What are you making happen in reality?

– What words did you not realize were words?

– Do you correct people not knowing if they are right or wrong?

– What do you know about history?

– What kind of storms have you been in?

– Do I have writer's block?

– Do you get writer's block?

– What causes writer's block?

– Why is it called writer's block and not something else?

– How tired are you right now?

– Can you even focus?

– Does it matter where one buys a cowboy hat?

– Where do you like to celebrate your successful accomplishments?

– What have you been talking about lately?

– Was I my sons last thought before he died?

– Did my son see happy memories of him and I right before he passed away?

– Shall I dedicate this second book to him?

– Will I also do a poem for his life or his death?

– Is death something morbid to you?

– Are you okay talking about death or does it make you uncomfortable, why or why not?

– Are you stuck in auto pilot and does auto pilot mean repetitiveness (same thing every day)?

– How are you going to get unstuck?

– Do you like a schedule?

- Have you ever had a picnic on a trampoline?

- What's your ideal date?

- What are you impressed by?

- What wild animals do you want to see up close and personal?

- Is what you do rare, why or why not?

- When will you set yourself free?

- Do you continue to use the same decorations for the holidays or do you always buy new ones every year?

- What have you forgotten about lately?

- Have you ever been requested by the court system?

- What are you feeling at this very moment?

- Have you ever felt like a failure and if so, how did you overcome it?

- Does music inspire you?

- Do you enjoy taking yourself out on dates?

- What's your light out of the darkness?

- What is your beat to the drum?

- How do you play your music?

- How do you relax?

- Are you patient, why or why not?

- Who's your shining star?

- What is your biggest complaint?

- What compliments do you give out?

- Do you trust yourself?

- What are you unsure of?

- What are you getting further and further away from?

- What walls have you put up?

- What gets lost in the stars or does it?

- Do you get lost in the stars?

- Do you hesitate on things?

- Do you show up early even when you don't mean to?

- Do you stall due to fear?

- What does courage mean to you?

- How many lives have been lost?

- Do you celebrate the living?

- Where do we go from here?

- What kind of vibes do you get from the places you go to?

- How well do you handle sorrow?

- When's the last time you gave someone flowers?

- Are you excited about the future?

- Are you holding onto the past?

- Are you stuck?

- Do you like watching the snow or rain fall?

- What's been stopping you from starting your own business?

- What are your luxuries and how long could you go without them?

- What helps clear your head from all that clutter?

- What have you put down and not picked back up for a while?

- Have you ever seen branches fall off of a tree and if so, did you enjoy the noise that the branches made during the whole process?

- Have you ever watched a water droplet on a window?

- What's the longest you've stared at something?

- Are you okay with what you're going through?

- How long could you go without your phone?

- Have you ever gotten sober and are you still sober, what's it been like for you?

- Where do you find the most peace?

- Can havoc create a sense of wholeness?

- Where are your pains and do you have a healthy way to get them to go away?

- What's the longest that you have ever been stuck in traffic?

- Knock knock…. Who's there? Knock knock…. Who's there? Knock knock…, me down will you ever get back up again?

- What trips you out?

- Where do you like to write the most?

- Are you considered stable?

- What does stable mean to you?

- Can you walk a straight line with your eyes closed and not run into things? FYI do safely please:)

- What do you not know that you're trying to understand?

- Do spirits feel cool or hot with in the fluctuation of the temperatures?

- Do you ever get hung up on one person or one thing in life?

- Could you meditate somewhere you've never been where there is a lot going on?

- If you were to die tomorrow, would you be happy with everything you did the day before and okay with what you posted last on the web?

- Do you wish you were a little kinder every day?

- Do you want to be more loving?

- Would you talk to God the way you talk to people or talk to people the way you talk to God?

- How many times have you changed in your lifetime?

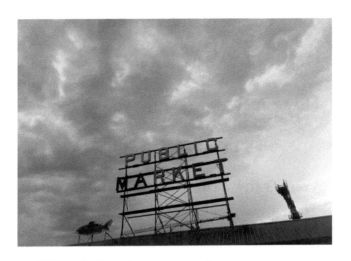

– What's foreign to you?

– What does purple mean to you?

– Have you been learning from what you've been reading?

– Did you know that there is heated clothing?

– What music do you listen to?

– Have you ever sat and looked at frost?

– What do you find interesting?

– Can you sit and listen to someone?

– Do you have a hard time sitting still?

– How much do you love you?

– Are you kind in traffic?

– What's the worst that could happen?

– Are you doing your best?

– What could you be doing to get things to be better?

– Have you ever sat and only watched geese?

– Have you ever watched a wild fox or coyote?

– Can you sit still?

– What does stillness mean to you?

– What sparks your inspiration, do you know?

– Have all of the leaves fallen yet?

– Have you ever seen fish eggs?

– Have you ever had fish that have laid eggs?

– What's it called once a fish has laid the eggs?

– Do you do poetry?

– What's the last poem you read?

– What is your favorite poem?

– Are you reserved about yourself and what you do in your life?

– What do you consider to be accessible in life and not accessible in life?

– What have you not worked on in a while?

– Have you ever watched a puddle, what did you see?

- Do you like looking at reflections?

- How many different types of salts are there?

- What's your name mean to you?

- What do you hear around you right now that is soothing?

- What words do you see around you and how many are there?

- How many sounds are around you?

- Who have you waited for lately?

- Are you a forgiving person?

- Do you know that you are loved?

- What's special to you?

- What interests you the most?

- How have you handled being let down?

- How well is your positivity holding up with everything around you?

- Do you like ice?

- Have you ever eaten the snow?

- What do you look forward to?

- What can you wait to finish up with?

- Can you smile at a stranger and still be, ok?

- What drives your bad behavior?

- What motivates you to be good?

- How long have you stayed up?

- Can you see the unseen?

- Do you seek out the unseen at times?

- Do you know that you are safe?

- What does be safe mean to you?

– What does removing mean to you?

– What results are you waiting for?

– Do people think your spiritual?

– How grounded are you?

– What is different this time for you?

– How many keys do you have let alone carry around with you?

– Does coffee wake you up or make you sleepy?

– Are you okay with vibrations of any kind?

– What's been helpful in your life?

– Who has been helpful in your life?

– What questions would you have for me if you ever met me?

- What kind of training have you had and what other kind of training do you want to go through?

- What have you responded to lately?

- What's the busiest you've ever been?

- Where do you see yourself going from here in your life?

- What does symbology mean to you?

- How many symbols do you see around you right now?

- How many symbols do you see in a day?

- What's your favorite symbol?

- What calander do you go by?

- How much coffee gets wasted?

- Can you enjoy the present moment?

– Have you ever played Xbox without the volume?

– Do you have a favorite hoodie?

– Do you open up your home to anyone?

– Do you accept all gifts that are given to you and really appreciate them?

– What do you find beauty in?

– Do you find beauty within yourself?

– How do you define beauty?

– Are you okay with your stomping grounds?

– Has anything disturbed your peace lately, what was it and do you think you can work through it?

– Are you good at swimming?

– Are you good at drawing?

– What are you practicing right now to be good at?

– What makes your heart jump?

– Where's your clarity?

– Do you like things to be clean?

– What does clean mean to you?

– What's your favorite instrument?

– What does flawless mean to you?

– What would be the perfect holiday for you?

– How would you like to get to know somebody?

– Are you comfortable?

– Are you doing something with your life and what might that be?

– Are you okay with how strong you are?

- What colors do you think the world could go without and why or why not?

- What could be better?

- What do you want to stop happening in your life and in the world?

- What animals speak to you the most and do you know why they speak to you?

- Do you believe in trolls?

- What opportunities are you taking a part in?

- What's the longest bath you've taken?

- Whose phone call do you avoid?

- Who are you gifting gifts to this year?

- Do you know that gifts don't have to be materialistic?

- What have you found lately?

- What have you rooted out lately?

- How do your tree roots spread?

- Do you like coffee beans?

- Do you know anything about where you live?

- What spirals in your life?

- Can you walk in a spiral?

- Can you walk a spiritual life?

- What is your mission?

- What is steady in your life?

- Can we help each other out?

- Can you count all the colors that are all around you right now? / How many are there?

- Can you inspire yourself?

- Do you know that you're a miracle?

- Are you hopeful?

– Do you care if people like you or hate you?

– Are you inspired at all times?

– What did you do this morning?

– Do you send out cards on holidays?

– Do you like to try new things?

– Do you do the same things every day, sticking to a routine?

– How do you mix things up in your life?

– Do you like to play in the dark?

– Who's your favorite writer?

– What light setting do you like?

– What kind of mood are you in right now?

– Are you truly happy?

- What scares people the most?

- Black or silver?

- Grey or white?

- Red or blue?

- Spray paint or oil paint?

- Acrylic paint or watercolor paint?

- Original or copy (print)?

- Pen or pencil?

- House or cabin?

- Apartment or studio?

- Cat or dog?

- Fish or birds?

- Being alone or being in a relationship?

- Bed or couch?

- Soft or firm?

- Sexual or sensual?

- Seductive or caressing?

- Chatty or reserved?

- How do you define you?

- How would you describe the ones you're around at this very moment?

- Do you believe that those we hang around define our very own character as a person?

- Who do you idolize?

- Who do you want to meet?

- Are you sexual?

- Where do you draw the line if any at all?

- What would life be like if there were no reflections?

- Can you see art in anything?

- Are you in any pain?

- What do you sneak around and do?

- Have you ever listened to the snowfall?

- Have you thrown a snowball?

- Have you ever built a snowman?

- Have you ever built a snow fort?

- Have you ever made a snow angel?

- What's colorful to you?

- What brightens up your day?

- How many pillows do you have?

- Carpet or hardwood floors?

- Ocean or river?

- Current or wave?

- Smooth or reckless?

- Clarity or spontaneous?

- Surprise or routine?

- Clutter or clean?

- Organized or distributed?

- What does organized look like to you?

- What does organized mean to you?

- Who do you have your lights on for?

- Do you cry in secret?

- Do you show anyone your silent tears?

- Are you a priority in your own life?

- Are you able to make yourself happy?

- What did you do to end the old year and bring in the new year?

– What's the sparkle in your eye?

– Do you like to color?

– What's your favorite moment or moments?

– Can you not work and take a day to yourself?

– Are you indirect or direct?

– What does make it in life mean to you, let alone look like to you?

– Are you able to sleep?

– Have you ever hyperventilated before?

– What makes your anxiety flare up?

– What gets your PTSD flared up?

– Are you eating, okay?

– What's the longest time that you have been on crutches?

– Do you accept help?

– Are you okay when you lose things?

– What do you do when someone steals something of yours?

– Have you ever had anything stolen?

– Have you ever stolen?

– What is your definition of stealing?

– What do you consider to be profound?

– Who do you consider to be spiritual in your life?

– Who do you vent to the most?

– Who or what knows you fully?

– How would a pacemaker work in outer space?

– Would you go into space given the opportunity?

- What new ideas have you come up with lately?

- Art you artistic?

- What do you wish you could do?

- Would you reread all these questions?

- What do you visualize?

- What do you work towards when you visualize?

- What do you do that serves you?

- Are you doing things that are healing?

- What's the most unbearable secret that you've ever had to withhold from someone?

- What's your medicine spiritually?

- What do you drink?

- What do you soak up mentally, emotionally and spiritually?

- Do you feel like you're a warrior?

- How do you feel about your spirit?

- How much time do you think you have?

- Are you going to build up or break down?

- Does the sunshine inspire you?

- What is your true nature?

- What is your maker to you?

- What do you see when you look at the sky?

- How do you praise what you believe in?

- Is there strength in one or is there strength in numbers?

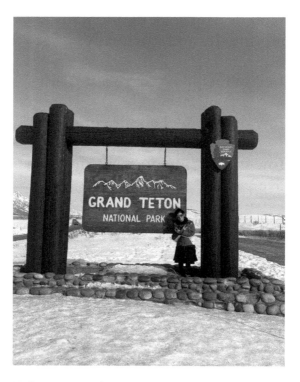

– What is it that you need?

– Who would you want to see again,
  alive or dead?

– What are you hanging onto that you
  should let go of?

– What has gone away that you wish
  would have stayed?

- Do you pick flowers or let them grow?

- What do you see in the future?

- What are your thoughts on what has changed in your life lately?

- What sparks your tears?

- Guitar or piano?

- Fighting or letting go?

- Giving in or giving up?

- Who needs you?

- What have you been dreaming about lately?

- What's been passing you by lately?

- What opportunities have you grabbed ahold of to produce a better life for you and others around you?

- Will I ever make it as a writer?

- Should I change what I do in my life completely?

- What animal do you relate to the most?

- Do you feel caged in?

- How free do you want to be?

- Do you like to doodle?

- Are you dense at times or do you even recognize it, and do you do your best to learn from it?

- What are your sometimes that you do?

- What are you in between right now?

- Can you look people in the eyes?

- Can you do public speaking?

- What is your throne?

- Have you ever been knocked over?

– Has anyone ever whispered in your ear before, do you remember what it was and if so what was it?

– Do you have any gems in your life?

– Do you cast sorrows or happiness with the words you speak?

– Do you show people everything that you're working on or tell them everything that you're doing?

– What is it that you're keeping to yourself that you're working on right now?

– Can you breathe slow?

– What is it about life that keeps you from wanting to live it?

– What your souls guide?

– Does music inspire you at times?

– Is your vision dead?

- What wounds are you healing right now?

- What memories would you want to hold onto forever?

- What are you insistent on?

- Is your soul at peace?

- Do you like to climb?

- Would you rub salt in your wounds if it meant that you would heal from them?

- What is it about society standards that's holding you back from doing what you want to accomplish?

- What are you discovering?

- What's by your feet and is it what you want in your life?

– Has anyone ever followed you
  through echoes of your life
  or spiritual essence of your
  steppingstones?

– Have you ever asked for forgiveness?

– Do you except where you are in your
  life?

– Are you ready to move forward with
  action and if so, what steps are you
  taking to do so?

– What do you do to get ready for bed?

– What do you do to get ready for the
  day?

– How do you pray?

– How do you meditate, and do you
  invite others to join?

– What roads have you yet to travel?

– Are you willing to treat yourself better as well as those around you including animals as well as plants and materialistic things?

– What does greed mean to you?

– Have you ever sat and played with a cat?

– What have you drawn lately?

– Do you want to leave?

– What's the meanest song you've heard or the one you listen to?

– What does soft mean to you?

– What is gentle defined by you and no one else?

– What do you want to fail?

– Have you ever seen anything explode?

– What does be upbeat mean to you,
 let alone look like to you?

– Do you like the smell of cinnamon?

– Do you wear rings?

– Do you put in the work?

– What battle is your soul in right
 now?

– What have you been asking for
 lately?

– Are you you rising up today?

– Do you listen to music with
 headphones on?

– Demons, do you believe in them?

– Can you withstand your own storms?

– Can you withstand your own
 sunshine and rainbows?

– Do you love what you were born with?

– Are you happy to be almost done or does finishing things scare you or make you a bit nervous?

– Did you know that it's okay to feel your feelings and that they won't last forever?

– What are facts in your life?

– Do you look towards your ancestors for wisdom?

– When's the last time you played like a child?

– Have you sat in front of a fire lately?

– Have you been playing any games with your friends lately or has it all been serious stuff?

– Have you ever been in a cave?

- Do you learn from the animals as well as nature?

- What do you consider to be a friend?

- What does friend mean to you?

- What are you excited about lately?

- Do you feel welcomed home let alone the places that you go to?

- What pathways would you not walk down on?

- What will you not do in life?

- What did you say you would never do and well some how you ended up doing it any ways?

- What would you erase from your life?

- As this comes to a close, has it been helpful to you, how so?

– Would you if you got a chance to meet me be glad you did?

– Is it better to go the extra mile?

– How can one better understand the other?

– Are you ready to let go yet?

– What have you picked up recently?

– What broke you into pieces?

– What do you think made you not enough?

– Do you like your own heartbeat?

– Have you ever listened to someone else's heartbeat?

– What do you dislike right now?

– Where do you hang your crown at night?

– What does inspiration mean to you?

- Did you know you create change not only in your life but also in others as well?

- What are the ripple effects in your life?

- Are you done settling?

- What does calm mean to you?

- Stillness or ripples?

- Boiling or calm?

- Walking or standing still?

- Do you share what you have?

- Do you fly, or do you soar in life?

- Gliding or skipping?

- Losing touch, is this something that you've done before or currently doing?

– What is it in belief that helps us to have a better quality of life?

– Are you raising hell here on earth?

– Do you like the magic that presides in all things that surround you?

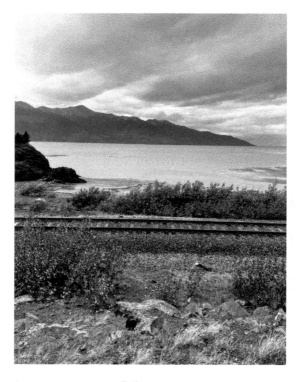

– Are you grateful?

- Have you found out your truths yet?

- What's your favorite song?

- What was/is your favorite cartoon show?

- What is your favorite show?

- Is your mind opening up more?

- Are you singing and dancing yet?

- Are you having feelings that you don't want to go away?

- Have you found what you've been looking for?

- What's been spinning in your life?

- What seems impossible in your life?

- Where's your light at?

- Have you ever been to the woods at a beach?

- Have you ever danced amongst the stars?

- What have you walked barefoot on?

- What do you look forward to?

- What do you see for you to do next in your life?

- What's caught your attention?

- Have you ever been buried in the sand?

- What does one day mean to you?

- What do you say thank you for?

- What are you waiting for?

- Do you use a computer for most of your day?

- What's personal to you?

- Have you ever played with your own shadow?

– Are you getting caught up in the better things in life?

– Do you give credit to your creator?

– What fears have you overcome recently?

– Do you feel accomplished yet?

– Would you give it all up for love?

– What does structure look like to you?

– Are you learning anything new right now and if so what is it?

– Do you feel safe?

– Have you ever felt lifted?

– What does soundness of mind mean to you?

– What does be lucky mean to you?

– Do you feel comfortable in your own skin?

375

- What's one thing that you've created that you're happy with?

- If the sky started falling down what would you do?

- If your story started to fall apart, how would you handle it differently this time?

- Are you standing tall for you or someone else?

- Who is brave in your life?

- Do you talk to animals, and do you listen to them?

- How do you relax?

- Do you share your story?

- Do you jump in rivers and enjoy the waters?

- Do you appreciate your story?

– Do you want to stay where you're at right now?

– How free are you?

– What colors do you wear the most of?

– What do you take the most photos of?

– What habits have you quit lately that you didn't think you would ever quit?

– Have you started anything healthy today or in the last month?

– When's the last time you've sat under a tree to enjoy it's s company and shade?

– Have you read a magazine recently and if so, what one was it?

– Will this book sell more copies then my first one?

– Did you enjoy the first one?

- What's been your consequences recently?

- Are you trying to cover up your heart or your soul?

- Do you feel fulfilled?

- What are your doubts right now?

- What's holding you back?

- How do you help yourself to get back up?

- How well do you handle not being in control?

- Can you truly let it go and just let things be?

- Have you ever been stranded?

- Have you been in a flood?

- Have you ever felt like you've been drowning?

- Have you ever drowned?

- What situations scared you the most?

- What situations surprised you the most?

- What situations helped you out the most?

- How do you learn the best?

- Are you learning at your best abilities?

- What are you lacking?

- Turning it over means what to you?

- What is your bright spot of your day?

- What bones have you broken?

- What's in your pocket that you always carry around with you?

- Have you ever been shell hunting on the beach?

- Where would you not get a tattoo?

- Where would you not get a piercing?

- What body modification would you do or not do?

- If you're given the chance, could you help end someone's pain stop forever, who would it be why or why not?

- Does having a broken heart really make someone stronger?

- Do you love your family, and do you feel as if those feelings are reciprocated?

- Do you believe that Mother Earth has her own mystical powers of healing as well as other powers?

- Do you believe music can be healing?

- How do you seek out ways of healing oneself?

– Do you believe feathers have healing properties as well as mystical powers too?

– What therapy if any do you seek out?

– Do you give back?

– What place do you find to be most peaceful to you?

– What does harmony mean to you?

– Do you ever hum to the sounds of Mother Earth?

– Does what you seek help your future or hinder it?

– How deep can you get emotionally, physically and spiritually?

– What does being broke mean to you?

– Where have you thrown your heart out to?

– How do you get your heart with it again?

– Does one seek inside or outside for peace or does one need both to be whole?

– Are you listening to positive things?

– What are you eating lately?

– Do you like the company in which you are keeping?

– How will this story end?

– What are your stories going to say at the end?

– Is it better to start at the end and work your way through?

– What does quality mean to you?

– How did you get here?

– What were you thinking that brought you to this point?

– Are you running away?

– Can I leave you with something positive?

– What does hydration mean to you?

– Is water life or is life water?

– What movement are you apart of?

– Can you sit and listen?

– Who is the wisest person?

– Have you ever heard a wolf howl in person?

– Have you ever prayed upon the waters?

– What does be resilient mean to you?

– Have you ever prayed to the trees?

– How deep do your roots go?

– How loud is your voice?

– Did you know you don't have to go it alone?

– How long can you listen for?

– What's the longest you've kept your eyes closed?

– What does hindsight mean to you?

– What are you like when you're feeling your feelings?

– What is your vibe like?

– What are your truths behind your energies?

– Do you know who believes in you the most and if so, are you surprised by those who do and for those who don't?

– Where do you shine your light the most?

– Are you okay with your failures and can you look them in the eyes while listing them?

– Well, what are they, are you ready to overcome them?

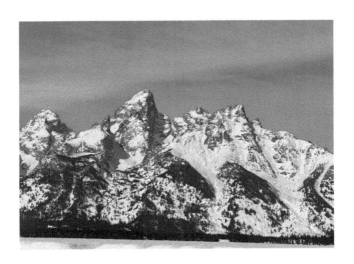

Unknowingly living life

Tearing in twenty million pieces,
Fallen in twenty-one million places,
Not knowing what are my phases,
Not knowing people's faces,
Carrying around a backpack, instead of
suitcases,
Around my whole body a blanket with laces,
Until your set free from the terrible places,
I will be covered and hidden from all other's
eyes and faces.

On the other side

Yes, my son has his disabilities,
As well as some difficulties,
Yet through his fantasies,
He can make it through the catastrophe's,
Through my dreams,
He's the way to be,
As the Great Spirit has shown me,
Happy and free.

Never let go of
life, just live

You may be feeling lots of pain,
Remember when you feel the rain,
That blood will always run through each and
every vein,
Don't ever let all your love get drained,
Just look up high and enjoy being sane,
In the Great spirits eyes no one is lame,
You may feel like you just got ran over by a
train,
Remember to always think with your heart
and not your brain,
That if you do, you'll only cause lots of strain,
Then shall nothing ever be the same,
Until the Great Spirit soon after lifts you up
just like a Crain,
To take you into his plane,
Where all things shall always forever remain.

The rose

A rose smells sweeter than
Anything in the air, or
Even anywhere,

The roses pedals are softer
then a rabbit's fur,

A rose with thorns hurts
When picked or handled
With or even touched by a
Small bug,

The stem of a rose is twice
The size of a Lilly or a Daisy,
The stem is a pretty green,
Until it hits winter days,

Roses come in all sorts of
Different colors and sizes,
Most everyone loves to have a
Dozen white roses sent to their door or
where-
Ever they maybe, they will always
Want a beautiful rose.

Getting through life's realities

My self-life was full of addiction,
 I had no affection,
   Only sorrow and aggression,
 To only live life with agitation,
     And getting stuck in an illusion,
For I thought I had lots of ambition,
      With people of association
       Only left me in confusion,
There was no benediction or benefaction,
      No such thing as compassion,
Which only got me into depression,
That led me more into consternation,
I'm going to give you a description,
Of what I need(ed) for my detoxification,
       One a lot of dedication,
       Some kind of devotion,
To ask for some help, by clarification,
        And I couldn't have done it without
my fiancé's inspiration,
       Oh, so awsome that we're so fusion,
    With our love, the way our
communication
      Always helps us with our love's connection,

So shall change our compassion,
As soon as this comes to a conclusion,
I just pray for more felicitation.

Alternatives

Life is crazy,
I'm so lazy,
   Wish I was a little hazy,
Smell'n like the sweetest daisy,
   I was slowly going crazy,
      Until you showed me that life has more,
      To be thankful for,
   You opened up the door,
Now I'm no longer bored,
So soon we won't be poor,
This was written in 2004.

Crazy, circled
journey of life

Look towards your life journey,
Are you still yearning to be learning,
Is there still turning,
Inside burning,
Or have you put out the fire,
In which things you desired,
Only then will you grow tired,
Nor will you longer,
Ever be any stronger,
So soon things get darker,
Where, there, evilness soon will Conquer,
Unless you grab for more,
Of the great paths,
Life door,
No longer shall you be bored,
Or even poor,
So soon people shall you adore.

Acid trip

You should never say goodbye,
You'll just drop down and cry,
Should you say hello,
You shall never be alone,
If you shy or say tiny white lies,
To your loved one's lives,
You must roll your dice,
For you'll always pay a price,
Then shall star nation reflect in your eyes,
So, hell becomes your only insides,
The demons, looking up at hells big skies,
You no longer own your heavenly moon lit
skies.

Walking down life's pathway not alone

Things seem like they were to plain,
Until you brought me to awake,
My family only led me to become insane,
You figured out that my smiles were fake,
Then you put icing on the cake,
Now you keep me on my tippy toes,
Never to forget my weary woes,
You showed me love, you showed me life,
You fly like the freest dove,
You showed me wrong, then taught me right,
But most of all you taught me how to stand up
and fight,
You tell me that I do not live into reality,
That all I've been going towards is insanity,
Then I knew that your heart had taken mine,
I hope your heart someday and you will lead
me towards the light,
To leave my sorrows behind,
So, we may just some time,
Someday intertwine.

Together or far apart, who broke our holy hearts

As I drink this glass of wine,
Smelling the trees of sweet forest pine,
Looking for you, I noticed there in a line,
For I hope you'll see I want you to be mine,
Can't you tell that as a pair,
Things are rough except smelling in the air,
Me being stubborn, yet just as soft as a bunch
of limes,
You as hurtful as a sunburn, yet just as strong
and protective as a bunch of knights,
That our lives have more meaning then ten
trillion, million and infinity of dimes,
Some days I wish that we were mimes,
Only cause of all of our stupid fights,
What's mine is yours and what's yours is mine,
That's what we use to say as friends with all
the good times,
It seems like we're always fighting,
Or just because we were always committing
some
Kind of crime,
We must work together to get some
communication.

Walking calmly

All that I need is some clarity and serenity,
So why don't you just stop with the profanity
and insanity,
Get back into reality,
Why not do some kind of charity,
Quit with all of the crime,
Cause you don't really know when it's your
time,
Close your eyes and count to nine,
Then see if you'll even be fine,
Why not walk that line,
See if you can even find a dime,
Keep walking on bye,
Don't stop for that graving of the glass of
wine,
Why not go to the restaurant and dine,
Stop and stay you should be just fine.

Disclosure for all these poems: they were written a long time ago in different relationships, different ways of living, and not in the best light of life. It has actually taken me a lot of courage to be willing to have these published into my book; my hopes are that, somehow, they will help others to live a better and meaningful life, not just for themselves yet also for those around them. Another disclosure: my son, Damien, has passed away. It's been twelve years since his passing. It happened while I was pregnant with my little girl. He was 5 years old. In March he would have been turning 18 years old. He was one of the sweetest and kindest sons a mother like me could have ever asked for. Damien, your smile and your laugh won't ever be forgotten. And my other hope is to let others know that you're not alone; no matter what you're going through, if you ask for help, it will be there. Peace be with all of you, and I hope you enjoy this journey, *On the other side of Ona a'o Nīnaus 2*, that it inspires you to accomplish your dreams too!

The end all done yeah!!!!!

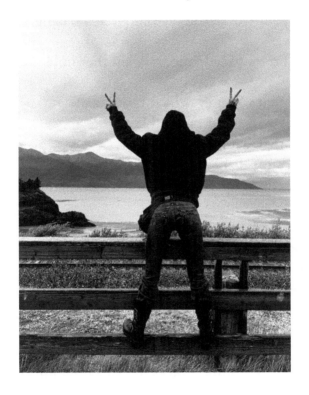

Since I saw you last

Those sweet blue eyes,
Wishing I didn't ever have to say those
goodbye's,
For your wonderful face and that amazing
smile,
Continues to help me walk another mile,

One that won't ever be forgotten,
The laugh that I can still hear,
Oh, my what life has brought,
We can feel and know that you are still near,
Thank you for your love and forethought,

My oh my have things changed in our life,
Sweet miss November has grown up so fast,
I'm no longer in a meager strife,
It seems as though life has zipped tight on
past,
As though you have only been gone for a fife,

Which November wants to learn the flute,
I've published going on now 2 books,
I'd like to believe you two would get along
and be very cute,

As brother and sister, you two definitely got
the looks,
You are a great big angel brother and thank
you for keeping
her safe and elocute,

We miss you and hope that you are flying with
star-nation,
For this we honor and ember you always!

About the Author

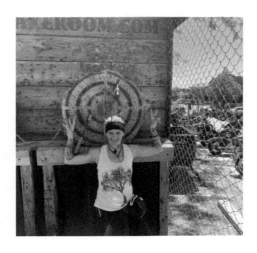

Megan Teraberry currently resides in Boise, Idaho where she is working on opening a business where she can offer art classes to the community. Her inspiration comes from all around her, and she believes she's open-minded to inspire creativity. Her beloved pets include her cat Yin and her fish in her 80-gallon tank. She enjoys traveling, painting, crochet, motorcycle riding, spending time with her beautiful daughter, and fishing. She feels immensely grateful for the great spirit, for without whom nothing in her life would be possible.

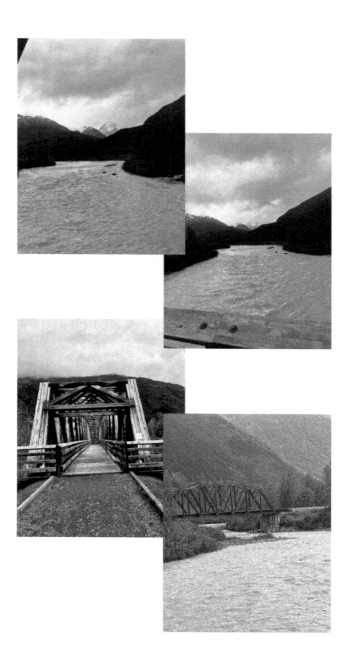

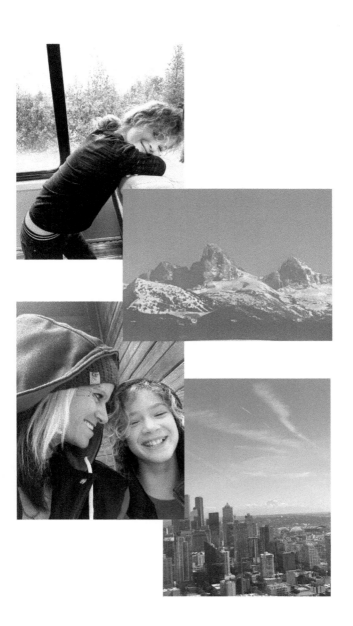

Milton Keynes UK
Ingram Content Group UK Ltd.
UKHW050252280324
440097UK00006B/27